PUT AN END TO YOUR TOSSING AND TURNING

This user-friendly resource offers a careful, step-by-step approach to discovering what's causing your sleeplessness. Learn surprising information on which remedies work and don't work, consider alternative methods to promote good sleep, and, most important, overcome your insomnia. Here's a sampling of the helpful, proven tips you'll find in this informative guide.

- Shop for foods that encourage peaceful sleep
- For women especially: know how hormones affect sleep
- Let exercise improve your ability to sleep
- Think again about that nightcap

Written in accessible yet authoritative language, this up-to-the-minute and inspiring book empowers you to find the answers and take action to end your insomnia.

INSOMNIA
50 ESSENTIAL THINGS TO DO

THERESA FOY DIGERONIMO is the author of several books on health and parenting. The coauthor of *Teach Your Child to Behave* and *Help Your Child Get the Most Out of School* (both available in Plume editions), she lives in Hawthorne, New Jersey. FRANK DIMARIA is a freelance and technical writer who lives in Clifton, New Jersey.

INSOMNIA

50 Essential Things to Do

Theresa Foy DiGeronimo
with Frank DiMaria

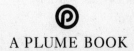

A PLUME BOOK

PLUME
Published by the Penguin Group
Penguin Books USA Inc., 375 Hudson Street, New York, New York 10014, U.S.A.
Penguin Books Ltd, 27 Wrights Lane, London W8 5TZ, England
Penguin Books Australia Ltd, Ringwood, Victoria, Australia
Penguin Books Canada Ltd, 10 Alcorn Avenue, Toronto, Ontario, Canada M4V 3B2
Penguin Books (N.Z.) Ltd, 182–190 Wairau Road, Auckland 10, New Zealand

Penguin Books Ltd, Registered Offices: Harmondsworth, Middlesex, England

First published by Plume, an imprint of Dutton Signet,
a division of Penguin Books USA Inc.

First Printing, June, 1997
1 3 5 7 9 10 8 6 4 2

Excerpt on pages 126–127 from Acupressure's Potent Points *by Michael Reed Gach. Copyright © 1990 by Michael Reed Gach. Used by permission of Bantam Books, a division of Bantam Doubleday Dell Publishing Group, Inc.*

 REGISTERED TRADEMARK—MARCA REGISTRADA

LIBRARY OF CONGRESS CATALOGING-IN-PUBLICATION DATA:
DeGeronimo, Theresa Foy.
   Insomnia : 50 essential things to do / Theresa Foy DiGeronimo,
with Frank DiMaria.
       p.   cm.
   Includes index.
   ISBN 0-452-27636-5
   1. Insomnia—Popular works. 2. Sleep. I. DiMaria, Frank.
II. Title.
RA786.D44   1997
616.8'498—dc21   96-53422
                                                                  CIP

Printed in the United States of America
Set in Caslon 540

To Mick, a very special night waker

CONTENTS

ACKNOWLEDGMENTS

I would like to acknowledge the help of the following people whose expertise has made this book as accurate and up-to-date as possible:

Donna Arand, Ph.D., Clinical director of the Kettering Sleep Disorders Centers, Kettering, Ohio

Sinan Baran, M.D., Sleep Disorders Center, Medical College of Pennsylvania and Hahnemann University, Philadelphia

Michael Bonnet, Ph.D., Wright State School of Medicine, Director Sleep Disorders Center, Dayton VA Hospital, Ohio

Brian Clement, Director Hippocrates Health Institute, West Palm Beach, Florida

Julia Cowan, L.M., Teaching staff director, Atlanta School of Massage

William C. Dement, M.D., Director of the Sleep Research Center, Stanford University School of Medicine, California

Brian Fradet, D.C., Madison Avenue Spine and Sports Medicine, New York

Cynthia Hetherington, M.L.S., Research librarian, New Jersey

Paul Hoagberg, Executive director of the Depression and Related Affective Disorders Association (DRADA), Baltimore, Maryland

Rochelle B. Mackey, R.N., C.N.S., M.A., Clinical director Mind/Body Medical Institute, Morristown, New Jersey

Jeffrey Nahmias, M.D., Sleep Disorders Center, Newark Beth Israel Hospital, Newark, New Jersey

Quentin Regestein, M.D., Director Sleep Clinic, Brigham and Women's Hospital, Boston

Annie Reibel, L.Ac., Plaza Center for the Healing Arts, Brooklyn, New York

Donn Posner, Ph.D., Behavioral and insomnia consultant for the Sleep Disorders Center at Rhode Island Hospital, Providence

Charles Schaefer, Ph.D., Director of the children's sleep-disorder clinic at Fairleigh Dickenson University, New Jersey

Sharon Schutte, M.D., Sleep Disorders Center, Thomas Jefferson University, Philadelphia

Anthony Spirito, Ph.D., Brown University School of Medicine Sleep-Disorders Clinic, Providence

Michael Stevenson, Ph.D., Clinical Director of North Valley Sleep Disorders Center, Mission Hills, California

Michael Thorpy, M.D., Director Sleep-Wake Disorders Center, Montefiore Hospital, Bronx, New York

Suzanne Woodward, Ph.D., assistant professor of psychiatry, Wayne State University School of Medicine, Detroit

INTRODUCTION

Trouble falling asleep or staying asleep—commonly termed insomnia—plagues approximately 70 million Americans of both sexes and all age, race, and socioeconomic groups. Although a common problem, insomnia is different from other ailments diagnosed by physicians because it is not a disease —it is a symptom much like a fever or stomachache. It takes a bit of detective work to trace the symptom back to the cause. Although a physician or sleep-disorder specialist may supervise this search, the real responsibility for uncovering the root of your insomnia falls to you. *Insomnia: 50 Essential Things to Do* is your code book. It will tell you where to look. It will help you uncover leads and rule out false clues. It will guide you through to a good night's sleep.

It's understandable why you're ready to put time and energy into your quest for solutions to your nocturnal problem. A recent study called *Sleep in America*, sponsored by the National Sleep Foundation and conducted by the Gallup Organization, found that insomniacs report significant impairment of daytime function and well-being, including:

- impaired ability to concentrate during the day
- memory problems
- difficulty coping with minor irritations
- impaired ability to accomplish needed tasks during the day
- less ability to enjoy family and social relationships
- feeling significantly less well physically

This book will help you find your way through the frustrating maze of insomnia. Based on information gathered from top sleep-disorder experts throughout the country, it will help you understand your body's need for sleep and the negative effects of sleeping pills on the internal cycles that promote a natural need for rest. It will take a look at common sleep zappers and help you zero in on the ones that may be robbing you of a good night's sleep. This book will teach you how to create a personalized sleep program, and it will share the latest research findings and treatment options. If all this fails to relieve the problem, you will learn about the programs and services offered by sleep-disorder centers around the country, and you will learn how to find and contact them. Finally, *Insomnia* gives you a wealth of reading material to help you pass the time during your sleepless hours.

CHAPTER ONE

LEARN MORE ABOUT SLEEP

#1

Learn What Happens During Normal Sleep

The average person spends about one-third of life in slumber. That means if you live to age seventy-five, twenty-five of those years will be spent asleep. Let's find out what happens during that time.

Before 1935 it was believed that sleep was largely static and filled with inactivity. But then the electroencephalogram (EEG), invented by Hans Berger, an Austrian psychiatrist, allowed scientists to record the electrical activity of the brain and determine that discrete brain wave patterns occur in regular cycles.

Today we know that humans experience two types of sleep: non-REM sleep (usually pronounced "non-rem" and written NREM) and REM sleep.

What Is NREM Sleep?

NREM sleep is normal sleep and is divided into four stages. During NREM sleep you lie quietly as your brain emits slow, regular waves. Depending on the amount of sleep you get every night, you can experience anywhere from four to six sleep cycles. Each cycle lasts about ninety minutes and contains up to four sleep stages and a REM period.

Falling asleep is like descending a staircase, with each stage of sleep becoming deeper than the previous one. At the onset of sleep you enter the first stage. This is a transitional period between wakefulness and sleep lasting only about three to five minutes. Alpha waves, emitted by the brain and associated with relaxed wakefulness, disappear and are replaced by slower, more regular theta waves. In addition, body temperature begins to drop and muscles begin to relax. Because some sections of the brain have fallen asleep and others are still awake during stage one, information from the environment is still being processed. Therefore, you are still easily aroused. It is not unusual for you to be awakened by a *myoclonic jerk*—a muscle contraction of the arm, leg, or entire body.

After the rather brief stage one transition period between wakefulness and sleep, you enter into the slightly deeper sleep of stage two. This sleep lasts about thirty to forty minutes. More time is spent in stage two sleep than in any other stage—about 50 percent of the night's total sleep time.

Stages three and four, the last two stages of NREM sleep, are usually grouped together. During these two stages brain wave activity slows down. Sleep becomes very deep as your brain emits high, wide delta waves. Because of the type of brain waves emitted, stage three and four sleep are often referred to as "deep delta sleep." Only 20 to 25 percent of the night's sleep is spent in stages three and four. Some children, however, can spend as much as 50 percent of the night in delta sleep. Growth hormone is released during stages three and four, making these stages very important for young sleepers. Stage four sleep often diminishes with age, sometimes disappearing totally in elderly sleepers. During stages three and four, heart rate and breathing become very regular. In addition, you become less sensitive to light and sound and are therefore difficult to awaken.

Delta sleep is valuable in restoring and revitalizing the body. When you are deprived of deep delta sleep, you often experience a feeling of uneasiness the following day. Delta sleep occurs during the first three hours of the night and disappears in the later sleep cycles.

After stage four sleep is complete, you ascend through stages three and two. Rather than going back into stage one and waking, however, you experience the night's first period of REM sleep.

What Is REM Sleep?

REM sleep is the period during which dreams occur. During REM (an acronym for *rapid eye movement*) your eyes move back and forth quickly beneath your eyelids as your mind dreams. (It is still unclear whether or not the rapid eye movements are a result of the eyes following the action taking place in dreams.) The first REM period of the night lasts about two to ten minutes. With each sleep cycle REM periods increase in duration. Brain activity during REM sleep is significantly different from the brain activity experienced during stages two, three, and four. During REM sleep there is activity similar to what you would see in wakefulness. While the EEG looks like the awake state, though, if you look at the muscle tone of the body, you'll find there is none. All skeletal muscle, with the exception of the diaphragm and the muscles of the eyes, are completely paralyzed during REM sleep. Researchers think that happens so people can't act out their dreams and hurt themselves. Indeed, when you are awakened during REM sleep, you are unable to move for several seconds until your muscle tone returns.

During REM sleep your heart rate becomes slightly irregular, and your breathing becomes very irregular, as you experience bursts of eye-movement activity and muscle twitches. Males of all ages experience partial or full penile erections, and women experience clitoral erections and an increase of blood flow to the vaginal area. These sexual reactions are usually unrelated to the content of dreams and reflect only the body's physiological state of arousal.

About one-quarter of the night is spent in REM sleep, and the majority of REM sleep takes place in the second half of the night. Each REM period becomes increasingly longer until toward the end of the night, they can last as long as an hour.

At the conclusion of the first REM period, the night's first sleep cycle comes to an end and you begin the second cycle of sleep. This cycle begins with stage two sleep and follows the same pattern as the first cycle. Once again you descend into the deepest stages of sleep and finish the cycle with a REM period. In adults, the later sleep cycles lack delta sleep. Stage four sleep disappears by the third cycle, and stage three sleep disappears by the fourth cycle. The last part of the night you alternate between stage two sleep and REM sleep. Because of the lack of delta sleep in the later cycles, the most restorative effects of a night's sleep are accomplished during the first three to five hours of sleep. It is not unusual to awaken after completing a sleep cycle. In most cases these awakenings are so brief that you don't even realize that you have awakened.

INSOMNIACS AND SLEEP CYCLES

This information about sleep cycles helps sleep researchers evaluate the severity of a person's insomnia. By monitoring sleep cycles, researchers have found that people with insomnia tend to overestimate how long it takes them to fall asleep and to underestimate how long they sleep.

Sleep recordings show that when chronic insomnia sufferers first fall asleep, they frequently alternate among stage one, stage two, and wakefulness. Severe insomniacs usually report that they were still awake when they are aroused from stage one—and sometimes from the early part of stage two. They appear to perceive the onset of sleep at a later time than other people, and they don't perceive themselves as asleep until they are well into stage two.

Dr. Arand says that some people go to sleep-disorders centers because they believe that they sleep poorly, only to find that objective physiological monitoring shows they sleep much better than they think. Sometimes this insight itself is sufficient to help them stop worrying about their sleep.

#2

FIND OUT IF
YOU ARE TRULY
AN INSOMNIAC

What is the magic number—the number of hours of sleep needed to rejuvenate the body and mind at night? Is it eight? Is it seven? Is it ten? The National Center for Health Statistics says that two-thirds of a population sample of 23,000 Americans over the age of twenty, including equal numbers of men and women, reported the need for between seven and eight hours of sleep. The number does not vary when comparing intelligence, mental health, or level of daily activity. Eight hours has become the standard by which normal sleep is measured. Even the majority of research subjects who live in darkened rooms without clocks spend one-third of their time sleeping.

SHORT AND LONG SLEEPERS

The problem with the magic number eight is that it fits the sleep patterns of only two-thirds of the population. This means that fully a third of Americans erroneously think there's something wrong with their sleep patterns. But in fact, about one in five healthy, non-insomniac adults sleeps less than six hours a night. (They're called *short sleepers*.) About one in ten sleeps nine hours or more (*long sleepers*). One person in twenty-five sleeps less than five or more than ten hours (a schedule followed by short sleeper Thomas Edison and long sleeper Albert Einstein). What these numbers say is simply: Sleep needs vary greatly from one person to another.

If you can't sleep a full eight hours every night, that doesn't mean you have insomnia. Maybe it just means you have something in common with a seventy-year-old nurse from western Australia who is a popular figure in sleep-research literature. It seems this woman answered a newspaper ad placed by sleep researchers Henry Jones and Ian Oswald looking for people who slept only a few hours at night. This subject agreed to be monitored in the sleep lab for one week. During this time Jones and Oswald found that this woman slept an average of only one hour at night. She took no naps during the day and showed no signs of tiredness. This subject said she had averaged only an hour of sleep since childhood. This is a striking example of why a person's sleep needs can't be dictated by standardized charts and graphs. There is no truly "normal" sleep pattern.

IS IT INSOMNIA?

Within each individual sleep needs remain quite constant. They change only very gradually over time. If we use the so-called "average" sleeper as an example, we find that sleep needs decrease from the time we're born, leveling to eight hours by age twelve, to seven hours between our mid-twenties and late forties, and dropping to five or six in our sixties and seventies. During each of these stages the amount of sleep you need one night is generally the same amount you need the next. There should be consistency in your sleep needs. That's how you know when there's a problem: when you can't get the sleep your body is accustomed to. If you've always required about seven hours of sleep per night and suddenly can't fall asleep and are getting only three or four hours of sleep, then insomnia becomes a serious consideration.

So, how much sleep do you need? Dr. James Perl, who has conducted a postdoctoral study of sleep and insomnia at the University of Colorado, says that you can judge how much sleep you need by evaluating your daytime alertness and energy level. If you feel wide awake, alert, and energetic throughout the day, you are getting enough sleep (even if it's only four or five hours). Dr. Perl believes that trying to sleep more is likely to create an insomnia problem when there was none to begin with.

If, on the other hand, you're consistently tired and irritable during the day, you can assume your body isn't getting enough sleep at night. If your tossing and turning is taking up needed sleep time, insomnia may be the culprit.

The questionnaire in Section 5 will help you map out your sleep history to determine if you're an insomniac or simply a short sleeper.

#3

INVESTIGATE WHAT HAPPENS WHEN YOU DON'T GET ENOUGH SLEEP

Most of us know how it feels to lose a night's sleep. The following day is filled with fatigue and irritability, and just making it through the workday is a major feat. Tasks usually easily accomplished become major dilemmas. Although lack of sleep surely does cause some problems, it does not have to be as bad as you think.

HOW DOES LACK OF SLEEP AFFECT THE BODY?

Research has indicated that performance does not diminish significantly until after about sixty hours of sleeplessness. "Other than being sleepy during the day, I think there are very few major effects that result from sleep loss. . . . For the most part, what people see as a result of sleep deprivation is very minimal and has relatively small effects," says Donna Arand, Ph.D., Clinical Director of the Kettering Sleep Disorders Center in Kettering, Ohio.

We can function and remain relatively effective on the days that follow sleepless nights because of the body's circadian rhythm or inner clock (see Section 38). The body's circadian rhythm is an important part of the sleep/wake cycle. It causes the core body temperature to increase to a peak and descend to a trough once every twenty-four hours. The body temperature of individuals who sleep during the night and are awake during the day begins to increase in the early morning just before they awaken. The temperature continues to rise until it peaks in the early evening. Alertness is maximum on the rising slope of the temperature curve, and sleepiness is greatest at the temperature's trough. When you remain awake all night, your circadian rhythm does not cease. Even though you are awake, your body physiologically and chemically is going through the same changes it normally would had you been asleep, says Dr. Arand. Because the body's circadian rhythm is a conditioned response, it takes about two weeks of sleep deprivation to alter the rhythm.

Individuals who have been deprived of sleep tend to perform poorly on tasks that are routine or boring like adding columns of numbers or entering data. They also have a tendency to dose off during sedentary activities such as watching television, reading, or driving. While performing more complex tasks, however, they make fewer mistakes and are less likely to dose off. Some experts believe that adrenaline provides the body with the extra boost it needs to make up for lost sleep.

During a period of sleep deprivation the effects of sleeplessness may become cumulative. So, the longer you are sleep-deprived, the worse your performance becomes. But once the body is allowed to fall asleep, the lost sleep can be made up in a surprisingly short period of time.

In the mid-1960s, a seventeen-year-old high school student named Randy Gardner attempted and succeeded in breaking the world record of 260 hours (almost eleven days) of sustained wakefulness. Gardner used no drugs, stimulants, or coffee during his feat. Members of the Stanford University Sleep Disorders Center monitored his actions carefully during his record-breaking attempt. They found that by the fourth day he had become irritable and had trouble concentrating; however, his mental and motor skills did not significantly deteriorate. In fact, after 230 hours of wakefulness, Gardner competed competitively against one of his friends and a sleep researcher in a hundred games of pinball, but was unable to recite the alphabet without mistakes. Toward the end of the study researchers noted that lack of movement and stimulation brought on extreme drowsiness, while activity restored him.

After Gardner broke the record by staying awake for 264 hours and twelve minutes, he went to bed falling fast asleep in just two minutes. He woke spontaneously fourteen hours forty minutes later and returned to his normal eight hours of sleep per night. Gardner's achievement showed that loss of sleep does not result in mental or physical breakdown and that lost sleep hours do not have to be paid back in full. The body has the ability to make up lost sleep efficiently because sleep that follows sleep deprivation is much deeper and of higher quality.

There are, however, some drawbacks to lack of sleep. You do feel sleepy. So if after you have been deprived of sleep, you plan to drive a vehicle or operate machinery that can cause injury, you need to exercise extreme caution or make other plans. Also, the World Federation of Sleep Society presented research in 1993 that showed that three hours or more of lost sleep per night can decrease the body's immune-system efficiency by as much as 50 percent. So it would be wise to avoid any situations that may expose you to bacteria or viruses on days when you had little or no sleep the night before.

#4

Identify Your Particular Type of Insomnia

There are three types of insomnia:

1. *Sleep onset insomnia* is characterized by an inability to fall asleep.
2. *Maintenance insomnia* is characterized by the inability to stay asleep.
3. *Early morning insomnia* is characterized by early awakenings.

All are lumped together under the heading insomnia. But each is quite unique in the way it affects sleep.

Sleep Onset Insomnia

Typically, the length of time it takes an adult to fall asleep is about eight to fifteen minutes. If you can't fall asleep after lying in bed for thirty minutes, you are experiencing sleep onset insomnia.

There are four basic reasons for this kind of insomnia:

1. Some people wrestle with their problems until the very last minutes of their waking hours. Even as they lie in bed, poised for sleep, their minds are occupied with matters, commitments, deadlines, etc. This mental wrestling match robs them of sleep.

2. Sleep onset insomnia is also a problem for people who have an extremely high energy level. These people are active until the very last minute of the day. When it is time to sleep, they are so wound up that the natural sedation necessary for sleep eludes them. Some people with high energy levels have high blood levels of activating hormones that are the result of glandular over-secretion, hyperthyroidism, for example. Stimulating drugs such as steroids can also cause hyperarousal.

3. The third cause of sleep onset insomnia is anxiety (see Section 11). Anxiety can be as severe as the terror that accompanies panic attacks or as mild as feelings of uneasiness. But at any level, because the body's physical response to anxiety is the opposite of how it reacts to sleep, it can chase away the calm of sleep.

4. The fourth cause of sleep onset insomnia is a stress-induced response to what is known as conditioned insomnia. Many people condition themselves to view their bed as a battleground. Not being able to fall asleep quickly causes such anxiety that their bodies are aroused to the point that sleep becomes impossible. This type of sleep onset insomnia is most often experienced by those who are accustomed to being in control of their lives. Often one night of sleeplessness

is perceived as a loss of control and can ultimately lead to sleep problems.

Maintenance Insomnia

Maintenance insomnia is experienced in the middle of the night about an hour and a half to two hours after falling asleep following the first sleep cycle. The inability to fall back to sleep after waking in the middle of the night can happen frequently throughout the night or only once. Usually awakenings that last less than seven minutes will be forgotten the following day. But several periods of awakening or one long period can cause tiredness and irritability.

There are several causes of maintenance insomnia. Aging, sleeping pills, certain medical conditions, alcohol, nicotine, and a sleep disorder called periodic limb movement disorder are all known contributors. How each of these causes maintenance insomnia is fully explained later in this book.

Early Morning Insomnia

Early morning insomnia causes people to wake one to four hours before the normal waking time. This type of insomnia is caused most often by depression. People who suffer from depression tend to experience frequent pre-dawn awakenings (see Section 10).

The environment of the room can be another cause of early morning insomnia. Factors such as light and noise can easily disturb a sleeper in the last four hours of sleep when sleep is not as deep. Sunlight coming through a nearby window or the sound of an early morning garbage truck can disturb a light sleeper. In these cases early morning insomnia can sometimes be "cured" by installing room darkening shades and by wearing ear plugs.

As you strive to identify and manage the cause of your

insomnia, fill out the questionnaire in Section 5 and the diary in Section 6. These will help you identify the time of night you have the most difficulty sleeping; compare this information to the three types of insomnia just described. This will help you identify your insomnia and will help you narrow down its cause and determine its treatment.

MAP OUT YOUR
SLEEP HISTORY

When people who have insomnia walk into a sleep disorders clinic, one of the first things they are asked to do is complete a questionnaire that will map out their sleep history. The following Sleep/Wake History questionnaire is part of the one that patients at the North Valley Sleep Disorders Center in Mission Hills, California, are asked to complete.

Although you don't have the insights necessary to make a diagnosis based on your answers to these questions, the answers will help you zero in on your sleep needs, style, and habits. This information will help you see what factors in your lifestyle may be contributing to your insomnia and which of the changes suggested in Chapter Two are most likely to improve your sleep.

SLEEP HISTORY

Usual Sleep Habits

Bedtime

My usual weekday (workday) bedtime is: .... _____

On weekdays (workdays) the *earliest* and *latest* time
in the last two weeks I have gone to bed is: .... _____

My usual weekend (off days) bedtime is: .... _____

On weekends (off days) the *earliest* and *latest* time
in the last two weeks I have gone to bed is: .... _____

To feel my best, I should go to bed at: .... _____

I frequently do not feel sleepy at bedtime and stay
up so late that I get little sleep: .... YES   NO

I have a job that involves shift work or night work: .... YES   NO

I frequently travel across time zones: .... YES   NO

I often sleep better in an unfamiliar bedroom, such
as a hotel or motel: .... YES   NO

Wake-up time

On weekdays (workdays) I usually wake up at: .... _____

On weekdays (workdays) the *earliest* and *latest* time
in the last two weeks I have awakened is: .... _____

On weekends (off days) I usually wake up at: .... _____

On weekends (off days) the *earliest* and *latest* time
in the last two weeks I have awakened is: .... _____

To feel my best, I should get up at: .... _____

I wake up naturally: .... YES   NO

　　　　by using an alarm: .... YES   NO

　　　　by someone calling me: .... YES   NO

Sleep Time

On average, how long do you actually sleep at
night?
   Weekdays (workdays): .... _____
   Weekends (off days): .... _____

How many hours should you sleep to feel your best? ... _____

How many naps do you average per week? .... _____

How do you usually feel after napping? .... _____

Sleep Onset and Maintenance

How many times in the past two weeks have you had
trouble going to sleep (sleep onset time greater
than twenty minutes)? .... _____

On average, how long does it take you to fall asleep? ... _____

My *shortest* and *longest* sleep onset time in the
last two weeks has been: .... _____

The number of times that I usually wake up during
the night is: .... _____

My best estimates of the clock time(s) during the
night that I wake up is (are): .... _____

If I wake up during the night, the time it usually
takes me to fall asleep again is: .... _____

The total amount of time that I am awake during the
night after I fall asleep is: .... _____

The dozing time that I spend between awakening in
the morning and getting out of bed is: .... _____

During the first thirty minutes after waking up in the
morning I usually feel:

very groggy .... _____
somewhat groggy .... _____
slightly drowsy, awake... _____
completely alert... _____

Insomnia

Use this scale for the following questions:
1 = never
2 = rarely
3 = sometimes
4 = usually

Do you feel you have a problem:

getting to sleep at night? 1   2   3   4
waking up during the night? 1   2   3   4
waking up too early in the morning?........................1   2   3   4
waking up too late in the morning? 1   2   3   4
feeling rested no matter how much sleep you get?...1   2   3   4

When falling asleep, or when just waking during the
night, how often do you:
have thoughts racing through your mind?.................1   2   3   4
feel sad and depressed? 1   2   3   4
have anxiety (worry about things)?...........................1   2   3   4
feel muscular tension? 1   2   3   4
feel afraid of not being able to get to sleep?............1   2   3   4
notice that parts of your body twitch or jerk? 1   2   3   4
experience restless legs (crawling or aching feelings
  and inability to keep your legs still)?....................1   2   3   4
  experience any kind of pain or discomfort? 1   2   3   4
  feel hungry or thirsty? 1   2   3   4

get awakened by noises?..1   2   3   4

get disturbed by your bed partner?........................:.1   2   3   4

find that heat or cold disturb your sleep? 1   2   3   4

have to urinate? 1   2   3   4

Daytime Functioning

For the following questions, refer to the scale
below and circle the number which best applies:

0 = asleep
1 = barely able to stay awake
2 = very drowsy
3 = a little sleepy
4 = awake but not alert
5 = wide awake and alert

How alert are you usually in the:

early morning? 0   1   2   3   4   5

late morning (midday)? 0   1   2   3   4   5

late afternoon? 0   1   2   3   4   5

evening?...0   1   2   3   4   5

night?...0   1   2   3   4   5

Use this scale for the following questions:

1 = never
2 = rarely
3 = sometimes
4 = often

How often:

do you feel alert and energetic the whole day?........1   2   3   4

do you feel overwhelming sleepiness (or struggle
to stay awake) during the daytime?..........................1   2   3   4

have you had problems with your performance at work (or school) because of sleepiness or fatigue? 1 2 3 4

have you been involved in automobile accidents or *near* accidents because of sleepiness or fatigue? 1 2 3 4

have others complained (spouse, boss, etc.) about your "laziness" or constant sleepiness? 1 2 3 4

do you find yourself falling asleep while reading, watching TV, or at entertainment events such as plays, movies, or concerts? 1 2 3 4

do you become confused or lose track of the topic during a conversation? 1 2 3 4

do you experience a sudden loss of muscle tone or weaknesses associated with an emotional experience such as laughter, anger, or surprise? 1 2 3 4

#6

START A SLEEP DIARY

A sleep diary can help you personalize your approach to beating insomnia. These diaries are a valuable tool used by most sleep-disorders centers to monitor the amount of sleep a patient is getting, the number of mid-night awakenings experienced, and the patient's perceived quality of sleep. Once you gather this information, it will give you some insight into your insomnia. In addition, if you decide to consult a sleep specialist, the diary will provide the feedback needed to assist you in improving your sleep. Dr. Stevenson of the North Valley Sleep Disorders Center in Mission Hills, California, says he encourages his patients to keep a diary of everything that happens in their life during their bout with insomnia. Keeping a diary can help answer questions such as:

- What has triggered the insomnia?
- What is causing it to linger?
- Is it related to a particular time of year or a certain night of the week?

• Do particular events in my life cause me to lose sleep while other events improve my sleep?

Keeping track of sleep time, wake-up time, and sleep quality can answer these questions and help you decide which kind of insomnia you have and what is causing it. Dr. Stevenson says that people who put a conscious effort into completing their diaries are the ones who experience the most improvement.

But bear in mind that keeping a sleep diary may cause you to pay more attention to your sleep than you should. Be careful! When you fill out your diary, step outside yourself and be as objective as possible.

The following sleep diary is adapted from the one used by Dr. Stevenson. He asks his patients to fill it out for seven to ten consecutive days. Give it a try—you may be surprised by what you find.

SLEEP DIARY

Date	Bedtime	Sleep Onset Time	# of Times Awake	Amount of Time Awake	Final Waking Time	Total Sleep Time	Sleep Quality	Notes

CHAPTER TWO

LOOK FOR THE ROOT OF YOUR INSOMNIA

#7

Kick the Caffeine Habit

Caffeine is a stimulant that has been called the insomniac's worst nightmare as well as best friend. After an awful night's sleep, caffeine picks you up and keeps you going. At the same time, it sets you up for another awful night's sleep. Thus begins the chronic cycle of tired days and sleepless nights. Whether caffeine is the root cause of your insomnia or just a contributing factor, your caffeine consumption needs to be addressed.

How Much Is Too Much?

Consuming more than 250 milligrams of caffeine before bedtime (two to three cups of coffee) will interfere with almost anyone's restful sleep; it increases the number of arousals during the night and reduces periods of REM sleep. Dr. J. R. Stradling, author of "ABC of Sleep Disorders" in the *British Medical Journal* says, "Because caffeine has a long half life (five hours), it is not just the coffee that is consumed in the evening that is important. Drinking more than six cups of coffee a day is likely to cause an increased number of arousals and insomnia." This is especially true for insomniacs, who seem to have a lower tolerance to the stimulating effects of caffeine than most people. Sensitivity to caffeine also often increases with age, so don't rule it out just because "it never bothered me before."

A COFFEE HUNT

Before you experiment with caffeine reduction, learn to keep track of how much caffeine you consume each day. (And don't forget to include headache remedies; they often contain caffeine.) You may be surprised by the total amount. The chart below will help you calculate your intake.

Item	Average Milligrams of Caffeine
Coffee (5-ounce cup)	
Brewed by drip method	115
Brewed by percolator	80
Instant	65
Tea (5 ounce cup)	
Brewed	40
Instant	30
Iced (12-ounce cup)	70
Chocolate bar (6 ounces)	25
Chocolate milk (1 ounce)	6
Coca-Cola	46
Excedrin	65
Dristan tablets	16

GIVING IT UP

The ideal solution to the caffeine problem is complete elimination. If you can give up caffeine, you'll be a giant step closer to licking your insomnia. Actually it's not that difficult today with the variety of decaffeinated coffees and herbal teas available. The biggest hurdle is breaking the addiction.

If you think you "just can't get through the day without coffee," you're probably right. Caffeine is addictive, and heavy caffeine users do need a morning hit and then another and another to feel alert. But once you clean caffeine out of your system, your body will once again be able to stay alert and function efficiently without those cups of coffee, tea, or cola.

When you first stop taking caffeine, you may experience withdrawal symptoms. You may lack energy or become sleepy during the day. You may be irritable, tense, or depressed. You may have headaches. For these reasons many people choose to eliminate caffeine gradually rather than all at once.

CUTTING DOWN

If you discover that caffeine is causing your insomnia but you can't give it up, that's progress too. At least you know what's keeping you up at night. Now, don't stop trying. Keep yourself on a very gradual withdrawal schedule. Switch to decaf later in the day; substitute a ginger ale for a cola; skip the second cup once in a while. Over time, as your body learns to do without repeat doses, you'll be ready to give it up completely.

Whether you give up caffeine all at once or gradually, the goal is the same: You want to awaken more alert in the morning and sleep more soundly at night.

#8

WATCH OUT FOR NICOTINE

"I'm going to have a cigarette and relax." This is a common statement but a biological impossibility. Nicotine, the drug found in tobacco, is a stimulant; it arouses and excites the nervous system. This explains why insomnia ranks high among the complaints voiced by smokers.

HOW DOES NICOTINE AFFECT SLEEP?

Nicotine can affect sleep in two ways. First, since nicotine is a central nervous system stimulant, it produces almost the same effects on the body as caffeine. Nicotine produces physiological arousal in the body that results in an increase in blood pressure, an increase in heart rate, and stimulation of brain-wave activity, all of which can affect sleep. Although at low blood concentrations nicotine may cause mild sedation and relaxation, at higher concentrations it leads to a state of arousal.

The second way in which nicotine may contribute to

insomnia is by interrupting sleep. Because nicotine is an addictive drug, it is craved by the smoker's body. This craving does not disappear during the night. As smokers sleep, their bodies go through nicotine withdrawal. This may cause smokers to awaken in the middle of the night craving a smoke. If a cigarette is smoked after a mid-night awakening, the nicotine will arouse the central nervous system and very likely will further aggravate insomnia, despite the initial mild sedation.

In experiments at Pennsylvania State University conducted by Dr. Anthony Kales, a group of men who had been smoking from one to three packs of cigarettes a day for at least two years stopped smoking. Dr. Kales found that despite displaying daytime withdrawal symptoms (temporary irritation, tension, fatigue, and restlessness), the men fell asleep faster at night and had less nighttime awakenings.

WHY SHOULD I QUIT SMOKING?

Your decision to quit smoking will make you less susceptible to a number of diseases. Every year more Americans die from smoking-related diseases than from AIDS, drug abuse, car accidents, and murder combined. Cigarette smoking is responsible for 20 percent of all the deaths in the United States. In women, lung cancer has surpassed breast cancer as the leading cause of cancer death. And now you have one more reason to kick the habit—the hope of getting a good night's sleep.

HOW CAN I QUIT SMOKING?

Breaking any type of habit is difficult—especially an addiction. There are several approaches and programs offered for the smoker who is ready to quit. The American Lung

Association offers these suggestions for those interested in quitting:

- Join a stop-smoking program such as Freedom from Smoking offered by the American Lung Association. This will allow you to meet other smokers who are also interested in quitting.
- Look into the various self-help options that are available. Freedom from Smoking and the American Lung Association offer guidebooks, videotapes, and audiotapes on kicking the habit.
- Pick a good time to quit. Do not choose a time when you know you will be under stress or when a holiday is approaching. Pick a date and tell everyone you are going to quit.
- Ask your doctor if a nicotine-replacement product (such as a nicotine patch or nicotine gum) is right for you.
- Keep a supply of healthy snacks on hand.
- Increase your daily exercise. Walk more.
- Make specific plans for what you will do when the urge hits. For example, take a deep breath, get up and walk around, call a friend, keep your hands busy. Remember, the urge passes in just a few minutes whether you give in to the temptation or not.
- Remove all cigarettes, ashtrays, matches, and lighters from your home, workplace, and car.
- Eat a well-balanced diet and drink plenty of water.

As you are trying to quit, you must remember that you are addicted to a drug. During the first few days after quitting, your insomnia may become worse. This is your body's reaction to the drug-withdrawal process. Don't get discouraged; the reaction is only temporary, and it will not be long before your sleep improves and you are a non-smoker.

Cigarettes are not the only nicotine-delivery system that affects a sound sleep. People who smoke cigars or pipes, or who chew tobacco or snuff, or those who inhale snuff through their nostrils, are also at risk of becoming addicted to nicotine and thus suffering chronic insomnia.

If you're a smoker and tired of losing sleep, you know what you have to do.

#9

Think Again
about That Nightcap

Some people use alcohol as a remedy for insomnia. In fact, that's why a drink before bedtime is called a nightcap. Because alcohol is a central nervous system depressant, many people are under the impression that it improves sleep. Actually the opposite is true. Alcohol is estimated to be the major cause of at least 10 percent of chronic insomnia cases. Alcohol initially promotes sleep. It has an initial sedative effect that leads to more rapid sleep onset. However, that is followed by arousals and sleep fragmentation later in the night. This results in an overall lower quality of sleep despite the more rapid onset.

Using alcohol to bring on quick sleep is a mistake. In addition to the fact that alcohol disturbs the quality of sleep, its ability to put you to sleep is only temporary. *The Pharmacological Basis of Therapeutics* by Goodman and Gilman reports that the rapid onset of sleep brought on by alcohol diminishes after three or more consecutive nights, causing insomniacs to continually increase the amount of alcohol needed to fall asleep. When they decide that alcohol isn't an effective remedy for insomnia and decide to give it up, they often experience a rebound effect, making it even harder to fall asleep.

WHAT ABOUT ALCOHOLICS?

The sleep patterns of chronic alcoholics are usually quite abnormal. They often experience disrupted, fragmented sleep not unlike the sleep patterns of people in old age. Chronic alcoholics tend to experience little or no deep delta sleep; they have decreased REM sleep and are plagued by frequent awakenings. These often result in complaints of daytime drowsiness. Alcoholics also tend to experience a more shallow sleep, a blurring of the wake-sleep rhythm, and also spend more time in bed. Even after chronic alcoholics give up booze, their sleep problems may not end. With alcohol withdrawal sleep can actually worsen and then ultimately improve in the long run. But the improvement may take months or even years.

Babies born to women who did not abstain from drinking during pregnancy also tend to exhibit abnormal sleep patterns after birth.

ALCOHOL AND SLEEP APNEA

Obstructive sleep apnea is a condition in which frequent and abnormal cessations of breathing occur, continuously interrupting sleep (see Section 40). The condition of sleep apnea can often be aggravated or initiated by alcohol. The sedative effects of alcohol cause the throat muscle to relax too much and also interfere with the involuntary awakening mechanisms. The condition of sleep apnea combined with alcohol use can become life-threatening, especially for those with a history of heart or lung disease.

When Can I Drink Alcohol?

If you have trouble getting a good night's sleep, you should not drink alcohol four to six hours prior to bedtime. A cocktail around dinnertime or a glass of wine with dinner will probably not remain in your bloodstream long enough to affect your sleep. If you have a problem limiting your evening consumption of alcohol, you may have a serious problem and you should seek professional help. Call Alcoholics Anonymous and ask for their questionnaire pamphlet; this will help you decide if you have a problem with alcohol that needs to be addressed before you can manage your insomnia. (See Section 50 for the phone number.)

10

CONSIDER DEPRESSION

It is often difficult to determine if a case of insomnia is caused by depression, or if depression is caused by lack of sleep. In many ways it is like the question "Which came first, the chicken or the egg?"

Helen, a woman in her late sixties, has a case of insomnia and pays her doctor a visit. She explains that she has not had a good night's sleep for the past six months. The doctor begins to take notes and asks if she has a bed partner that may be disturbing her sleep. "No," Helen says sadly, "my husband died suddenly of a heart attack last year." "Did you have trouble sleeping before your husband passed away?" asks the doctor. At this point Helen sees the connection. Her nighttime battles began shortly after her husband's death. The depression she has fallen into is the cause of her insomnia.

How Does Depression Affect Sleep?

"Insomnia is a very common feature of depression," says Dr. Sinan Baran from the Sleep Disorders Center at the Medical College of Pennsylvania in Philadelphia. "About ninety percent of the patients who are depressed have insomnia, and about ten percent have hypersomnia, meaning they sleep longer or more than usual."

People who suffer from depression tend to experience a less restorative sleep than those who are not. Depressives exhibit any or all of these types of insomnia: frequent predawn awakenings, less deep sleep, and diminished overall sleep time. By far the most common type of insomnia experienced by a depressive is frequent predawn awakenings. Paul Hoagberg, executive director of the Depression and Related Affective Disorders Association (DRADA), suffers from a bipolar disorder. Throughout his life he has experienced the highs of mania and the lows of depression; however, his more serious problems have stemmed from his depressions. He describes the insomnia that accompanied his depressive episodes in this way: "Falling asleep would be okay, but at two or three in the morning I'd be awake with just a terrible, terrible feeling. . . . F. Scott Fitzgerald, who I'm sure was a depressive and who of course medicated his depression with booze, once wrote, 'In the dark of the soul, it is always three o'clock in the morning.' A very good description." During his depressions Hoagberg would lose the ability to concentrate and would experience a constant feeling of anguish. He says it was as though he wanted to "run out of my body and get away from myself." His insomnia continued for the duration of his depression. Not surprisingly, when his depression eased, his sleep improved.

WHO SUFFERS FROM DEPRESSION AND WHAT ARE THE SYMPTOMS?

Statistically, women are about two times more likely to develop a depression than men. Depression is also more likely to surface in the elderly. Depression in the twilight years is usually related to chronic illness, which often can have a major impact on lifestyle. Chronic illness is believed to deplete the immune system, and therefore some experts suggest that there is a link between the immune system and depression. It is important for people who are sixty years and older and are experiencing insomnia to be screened for depression. Many doctors make the mistake of assuming that poor sleep in the elderly is due to old age. Although sleep does change with age (see Section 18), it should not be assumed that age is the only cause.

Depression is a continuous feeling; it's not just having one bad day. If you experience at least four of the following symptoms for a period of two weeks, you may be suffering from a clinical depression:

- persistent sadness
- loss of interest in most activities
- irritability or anger for no good reason
- feelings of worthlessness or uselessness
- desire to be alone and not to be bothered
- inability to concentrate or make decisions
- feeling slow, mentally or physically
- aches and pains that do not respond to treatment
- having trouble sleeping (particularly early morning awakening)
- sleeping too much
- loss of appetite or increased appetite

- using alcohol or other drugs in excess to feel better
- repeated thoughts of death or suicide

Dr. Baran believes diminished interest in activities that were once enjoyed is the clearest indication of a depression. This symptom, along with a persistently depressed mood, is what psychiatrists look for when evaluating a patient suspected of suffering depression.

What Are the Causes of Depression?

In most cases depression is caused by a combination of factors. Probably the most common cause is genetic predisposition. Two-thirds of depressed patients have family members who have suffered from depression. *The Diagnostic and Statistical Manual of Depressive Disorders* suggests that immediate biological relatives of depressed persons have a 15 percent chance of developing a depression, while grandchildren, nephews, and nieces have a 7 percent chance. People who do not have relatives who have suffered depression have only a 2 to 3 percent chance of developing the disorder. Even when children born to depressed parents are adopted and reared apart in a different household, they are three times more likely to develop a depression. Evidence of genetic predisposition is supported by studies of identical twins (twins who carry the same genes). It has been found that if one twin is depressed, the other has a 70 percent chance of developing the disorder—even when the twins are reared apart.

Genetic predisposition is not the only cause of depression. Events and experiences such as chronic medical illness, loss of a loved one, loss of a job, retirement, problems in relationships, unresolved grief, suppressed anger, helplessness, and drug and alcohol abuse are all factors that can cause depression.

How Is Depression Treated?

There are a number of lifestyle changes you can make to improve your chances of beating a mild depression. Let's take a look at five:

1. Because depression becomes worse during times of inactivity, you may want to establish a routine that includes some form of exercise (see Section 37). Physical activity can help improve your state of mind as well as your physical health.
2. Take time out to participate in activities that you enjoy. If you like going to concerts, do so on a regular basis.
3. Try to identify the possible sources of your depression and if possible avoid them.
4. Don't be so hard on yourself. Rather than focusing on the negative aspects of your personality and appearance, identify and focus on the positive ones.
5. Join a self-help group. It will give you the opportunity to discuss your problems with a sympathetic listener. For more information about self-help groups in your area, call the Depression and Related Affective Disorders Association (DRADA), listed in Section 50.

For depressions that are more severe, you should seek help. Professional treatment is effective for more than 80 percent of depressed patients. If your physician prescribes drug therapy to treat your depression, be aware that many drugs come with a long list of possible side effects—including sleep disturbance. So if you find that your insomnia may be caused by depression, don't let the cure aggravate the condition. Talk to your doctor about your sleep problems and how they relate to your depression and its treatment.

#11

CHECK YOUR ANXIETY LEVEL

After recently taking his marriage vows, Walter returned from his honeymoon tanned, refreshed, and ready to begin life with his new bride. The first evening back, however, he had a difficult time falling asleep. The following night he had the same trouble. After several weeks of sleepless nights, Walter sought professional help. His doctor questioned him to find the root cause of his insomnia.

"How's work? Do you have any problems there?" his doctor asked.

"No. Everything at work is great. I love my job," Walter replied.

"Has anything unusual happened to you in the past month or so? Has there been any tension between you and a close friend or your wife?" asked the doctor.

"No. I love my wife. You know, we're only married about a month," Walter added.

"One month? Didn't you say you started having trouble sleeping one month ago?"

"Yes," admitted Walter, "but I'm happy with my marriage. Why would that keep me awake?"

Although on the surface Walter was happy, marriage brought with it a drastic change in lifestyle that resulted in stress and anxiety—and insomnia. There are many life situations and emotional circumstances that can cause sleepless nights. Some are rooted in simple, everyday stress, others in anxiety, and some others in the more serious anxiety disorders.

WHAT IS STRESS AND WHERE DOES IT COME FROM?

Stress is the body's response to circumstances that seem threatening or challenging. Events and situations that you perceive as threats or challenges are called stressors. These can be positive events, like starting a new job, getting married, or becoming a parent. Stressors can also be negative events, like dealing with an irate boss, getting stuck in traffic, or undergoing surgery.

WHAT IS THE BODY'S RESPONSE TO STRESS?

Our response evolved long ago to give the species a better chance of survival. Prehistoric man faced a variety of stressors much different from the ones we face today. He was not likely to be laid off from his job, or be involved in an automobile accident, but he might have faced the problem of being unable to find sufficient food for his family, or of being preyed upon by large animals.

When prehistoric man was confronted by a predator (probably his most feared stressor), his heart rate would increase, his muscles would tighten, his breathing would become shallow and quick, adrenaline would be released, and he would begin to perspire. An increase in the activity of the nervous system was preparing him for physical exertion during "fight or flight." After the altercation the nervous system returned his body's functions to their normal levels. This automatic stress response of our predecessors is still active in us today.

Your response to stress is the same as your ancestors. But unlike prehistoric man, you have far fewer ways to release the energy produced by the stress response. Therefore, much of the energy is turned inward and can result in distress, stress-related illnesses, and in some cases insomnia. As the stress level goes up or as anxiety increases, one is more prone to sleeplessness.

WHAT IS ANXIETY?

Anxiety is the experience of fear and worry. Although anxiety has been around since the beginning of time, it was not until 1844 that it was described and given a name by the Danish existentialist Soren Kierkegaard. Feelings of anxiety may be experienced with no apparent external stressor—it may simply come from within. "People who are anxious often have a sense of some sort of impending threat or doom," says Donn Posner, Ph.D., behavioral and insomnia consultant for the Sleep Disorders Center at Rhode Island Hospital, Providence. "They will experience a host of physical symptoms that go along with that, which may include (but don't have to): a racing heart, shortness of breath, perspiration, jitteriness, shakiness, chest pains, tingling in the extremities, numbness in the extremities, dizziness, and light-headedness. These are all symptoms of anxiety."

Anxiety can be experienced at various levels ranging from mild feelings of uneasiness to the severe terror that accompanies panic attacks. In all, about 28 million Americans have diagnosable anxiety disorders.

Anxiety, as well as anxiety disorders, can affect your sleep. The physiological process of anxiety versus that of sleep are quite opposite. "We're looking at autonomic nervous system arousal in anxiety disorders," notes Dr. Posner, "and when we're sleeping, we're trying to relax and depress this same autonomic system. If you become anxious, you're moving your physiological system in the opposite direction from where it needs to go when you want to sleep."

It's true that too much stress can be a long-term risk factor to your health, but it's also true that without the hidden reserves of energy released by stress, you would not be able to make that big presentation at work. In fact, without some anxiety it would be virtually impossible to be productive. So don't try to eliminate all stress from your life. Rather, focus on the stress that interferes with your productivity, happiness, and sleep. Then try the relaxation techniques described in Section 36. If you continue to feel anxious, you should contact a mental health professional who can help you.

#12

FIND OUT IF
YOUR MEDICAL CONDITION
MAY AFFECT SLEEP

All medical conditions, from an irritating allergy to a life-threatening brain tumor, have the potential to interfere with sleep. Sometimes the symptoms of a medical condition seem only an inconvenience during the day but become a major irritant at night. Let's take a look at some of these conditions that can cause sleep disturbances.

RESPIRATORY DISORDERS

- Asthma, bronchitis, and emphysema all may interfere with breathing and cause nighttime arousals.
- Allergies can irritate eyes and the throat as well as cause a stuffed nose; these all interfere with sleep.
- Sleep apnea, a condition caused by anatomical problems such as an oversize uvula (the tag of flesh that hangs from the soft palate of the mouth) combined with the relaxation of the throat muscles during sleep, causes some sleepers to cease breathing from ten sec-

onds to three minutes (see Section 40). These apneic episodes often result in nighttime awakenings. Sleep apnea and its effect on sleep are sometimes exacerbated by the use of alcohol, sleeping pills, and obesity.

CARDIOVASCULAR DISORDERS

- Lack of oxygen to the heart muscle results in a condition known as angina, which frequently occurs during sleep. Some experts theorize that angina attacks are a response to the content of dreams, since most attacks occur during REM sleep. During an angina attack an individual may be awakened by a choking pain.
- Congestive heart failure can inhibit breathing, resulting in nighttime arousals. Sometimes as individuals lie in bed in the quiet of the night, they can hear their own cardiac arrhythmia (irregular heartbeats). This can be very unsettling, and this stress can lead to physiological arousals that prevent sleep.

DIGESTIVE DISORDERS

- Gastroesophageal reflux, commonly known as heartburn, is a condition in which the contents of the stomach, including the acid that is produced in the stomach, reflux or "back up" into the esophagus (the tube that connects the throat with the stomach). When this happens the esophagus becomes irritated and inflamed, causing a burning sensation that has the potential to awaken a sleeper. If you experience heartburn that wakes you in the night, you should avoid eating spicy foods and drinking alcohol, tea, coffee, and colas. Also, you should not smoke. It might help if you wait at least three to four hours after eating before lying down. Once the heartburn starts, try elevating the head of your bed or using pillows to elevate your head above the level of your feet. If your heartburn persists, see your doctor.

• An ulcer is a damaged portion of stomach or duodenal wall (part of the small intestine) exposed to gastric juices. Ulcers may be caused by excess secretion of gastric acid or pepsin or by deficient secretion of the gastric mucus that protects the stomach or duodenal from the gastric juices. When food leaves the stomach or duodenal during the night, the ulcer is bathed in acid. The resulting pain can cause a nighttime awakening. An estimated four thousand Americans develop an ulcer each day. If you think you may be suffering from an ulcer, see your doctor immediately.

BLADDER PROBLEMS

As the bladder fills during the night it contracts, resulting in lighter sleep and quite often an awakening. Michael Stevenson, Ph.D., clinical director of North Valley Sleep Disorders Center, Mission Hills, California, prescribes two exercises for his patients who cannot make it through the night without a trip to the bathroom:

1. Once a day drink as much liquid as you can. Hold the liquid in your bladder for as long as you can before expelling it. Increase the amount of liquid each day. This exercise conditions the bladder to delay urination.

2. The second exercise is called a kegel. Kegels are sometimes practiced by women during pregnancy to strengthen the muscles used during childbirth; it's also recommended to women having difficulty achieving orgasm and men who experience premature ejaculation. To perform the exercise Dr. Stevenson has

his patients sit in a chair and contract the voluntary muscles that restrict the flow of urine during urination, pulsating the muscles repeatedly twenty to thirty times. Then they contract the muscles and hold them tightly for as long as they can. Strengthening these muscles allows you to hold your urine longer without a nighttime run to the bathroom.

SKELETAL DISORDERS

People who suffer from rheumatoid arthritis or other similar disease of the joints often have trouble sleeping. A typical nighttime movement like rolling over can irritate the inflamed joints and awaken the sleeper.

PREGNANCY

Early in pregnancy (especially in the first three months) hormonal changes can affect an expectant mother's sleep. Progesterone has a sedative effect, often causing daytime drowsiness. This is often the first sign of pregnancy. Later in pregnancy, as the size of the fetus increases and its movements intensify, the mother's sleep is often disturbed by physical discomfort.

All of these medical conditions and many, many others can interfere with a good night's sleep. Before you blame your sleepless nights on insomnia, be sure to consider other medical conditions.

#13

CONSIDER THE EFFECTS OF YOUR OVER-THE-COUNTER AND PRESCRIPTION MEDICATIONS

When you are searching for the root cause of your insomnia, it may be a good idea to take a look in your medicine cabinet. Even the mildest over-the-counter drugs, as well as the more potent medications prescribed by your physician, can have a profound effect on sleep. Difficulty falling asleep, frequent interruptions during sleep, and early morning awakenings all can be a result of the medications you take.

Listed below are some drugs that have been known to interfere with sleep. Don't be surprised if you find the cause of your insomnia in a little bottle:

- medications containing caffeine such as Excedrin, Anacin, or Triaminic
- many antidepressant drugs
- some birth-control pills
- bronchodilating drugs for asthma that contain ephedrine, aminophylline, or norepinephrine
- steroid preparations

- some thyroid preparations
- Dopar for Parkinson's disease
- drugs containing adrenocorticotropic hormone (ACTH)
- some cancer chemotherapeutic agents
- sleeping pills and tranquilizers
- some drugs for high blood pressure
- prescription diet pills containing an amphetamine

That's quite a number of possible sleep disturbers! You may wonder why sleeping pills and tranquilizers are on a list of drugs that can cause insomnia. It's because once our body is conditioned to fall asleep aided by sleeping pills or tranquilizers, insomnia can result when you discontinue taking them (see Chapter 4).

WHAT CAN I DO TO PREVENT MY PRESCRIPTION AND OVER-THE-COUNTER MEDICATIONS FROM AFFECTING MY SLEEP?

If your doctor prescribes a medication that disrupts your sleep, you may want to ask her two questions. First, ask if there are other medications or treatment alternatives to the prescribed medication. If not, ask if the medication can be taken at a different hour of the day so it won't disturb your sleep. If you find a prescribed medication is disrupting your sleep, the effects may be temporary. If your sleep changes after going on a medication, check with your doctor. Sometimes side effects go away after the body adjusts to the new medication.

When you take prescription or over-the-counter medication, you should educate yourself on the possible side effects. Side effects of over-the-counter drugs are listed on the packaging. Prescription medications come with a package insert that lists possible side effects. If your prescription does not come with an insert, ask the pharmacist or your physician about side effects; you need to know.

Drugs do not affect everyone in the same way. Today many drug inserts indicate the possible side effects that can occur in the elderly as well as those that can occur in younger people. Also, a medication that causes drowsiness in one individual may cause insomnia in another. Do not assume that the side effects listed on a drug's packaging or on the package insert are definitely going to happen to you, or that they are the only possibilities. Ask the pharmacist and/or your physician if any of the ingredients are known to affect sleep.

If you are being treated by two or more physicians, it is important you tell each one about all medications you are taking. Sometimes a single drug may have no effect on sleep, but when it is combined with another medication problems can occur.

What About Illicit Drugs?

Marijuana. Marijuana exhibits characteristics of a depressant as well as a stimulant; however, it is classified as neither. Delta-9 tetrahydrocannabinol (THC), the psychoactive compound found in marijuana, alters brain chemicals involved in sleep and produces changes in brain-wave patterns. It has been documented that individuals using marijuana spend less time in REM sleep, but spend more time in stage four sleep. It should be noted that marijuana does not affect everyone in the same way. Some are stimulated while others are sedated by its use.

Amphetamines. Amphetamines, also known as crank or speed, are powerful stimulants that intensify the brain chemicals involved in wakefulness and produce changes in brain-wave patterns. Amphetamines reduce the stages of deep sleep and REM sleep. They also delay sleep onset, increase the chances of waking after sleep onset occurs, and decrease total sleep time. Withdrawal from amphetamines can lead to REM rebound (an increase in REM sleep), which is sometimes accompanied by nightmares.

Cocaine. Cocaine is a potent, addictive stimulant that produces a sense of euphoria only to be followed by a severe depression. Cocaine affects dopamine, a chemical in the brain that plays a role in motor coordination as well as sleep and wakefulness. Cocaine use produces insomnia caused by a reduction in deep sleep and REM sleep. Discontinuing the use of cocaine produces a sleepy feeling. Cocaine users often feel as though they need the drug to relieve themselves of the tired feeling and to function normally.

Heroin. The depressant heroin inhibits intellectual functioning and motor functioning. Heroin use causes a decrease in deep sleep and REM sleep as well as causing frequent shifts from stage one sleep to wakefulness. Discontinuing the use of heroin can lead to REM rebound that can cause nightmares.

It is up to you to investigate how the drugs you are taking may be affecting your sleep. The more you know about the ingredients in each medication, the easier it will be to determine if they are the cause of your insomnia.

#14

Take a Close Look at Your Daily Schedule

The human body needs regular periods of work, rest, and play. However, many of us lead lives that lack regularity and rhythm, and this can cause insomnia. If you want to get a good night's sleep, it's important to create a daily schedule that offers the body a predictable routine.

Thirty-eight-year-old Tom Sweeney is married, has two kids, and owns a small business. He also had insomnia for about a year. Looking for the cause of his sleep problem, Tom ruled out caffeine, nicotine, alcohol, depression, anxiety, medical conditions, and the side effects of medication. At a loss to explain why he couldn't sleep, he decided to keep a written record of his daily schedule. What he found surprised him. Tom had no regularity or routine to his days at all. Some nights he'd stay up until two in the morning and get up at ten; other nights he'd be sound asleep by nine-thirty and up at the crack of dawn. Some days Tom would take his daily jog before work; others days he'd run after dinner. Some days he ate three square meals; sometimes he barely stopped to shove a doughnut into his mouth. All Tom's activities happened in haphazard, random order. This, experts tell us, upsets the body rhythm and can cause insomnia.

What Is Body Rhythm?

Body rhythm is known as the inner clock or circadian rhythm. Circadian rhythm (from the Latin *circe*, meaning "about," and *dies*, meaning "a day") is an innate, daily fluctuation of physiological and behavioral functions including sleep and waking. These functions are generally linked to the twenty-four-hour light-dark, day-night cycle. Circadian rhythms are coordinated by small nuclei at the base of the brain called the suprachiasmatic nuclei (SCN). The SCN work with other parts of the brain to control the body's temperature, hormone release, and other functions. In most healthy individuals body temperature begins to rise during the last few hours of sleep just before they awaken. This rise in body temperature seems to promote a feeling of alertness in the morning. In the evening, body temperature begins to decrease in preparation for sleep. A dip in temperature is also experienced in the late afternoon between about two and four, which may explain why people tend to feel drowsy at this time. The naturally occurring circadian period is about twenty-five hours long in most individuals. If you had the opportunity to live in a world that was free of all morning commitments and alarm clocks, you would most likely find yourself rising and falling asleep one hour later every day. The more regular your schedule, the easier it is to retrain your circadian rhythm in a twenty-four-hour time period.

Keep Track of Your Daily Schedule

To train the body's circadian rhythm, you should put yourself on a daily schedule that promotes regularity, rhythm, and balance. Keep a written record for seven to ten days to record the time of repetitive activities like sleeping, waking, eating, and exercising. Then examine your schedule honestly. Does it give your body rhythm a consistent pattern? If not, try drawing up a daily schedule that fits your needs and still holds a repetitive rhythm. Activities like meals, exercise, naps, wake-up times, and bedtimes should be scheduled for specific times of the day and should occur at roughly the same time each day. Donn Posner, Ph.D., insomnia consultant for the Sleep Disorders Center at Rhode Island Hospital in Providence, suggests, "You should have the same number of meals and have them around the same time every day. If you're going to take a nap, program the nap and have it at a certain time of the day. When you exercise, exercise at a certain time of the day. These things teach the body what time it is and train the circadian rhythm."

SLEEP HYGIENE AND YOUR DAILY SCHEDULE

Sleep hygiene is lifestyle and dietary habits that promote sound sleep. Unfortunately, just practicing good sleep hygiene is not always enough to prevent insomnia. The daily scheduling of sleep-hygiene elements is important as well. "When we talk about sleep hygiene," says Dr. Posner, "we're talking about the effect it has on your body. For example, what effect does a snack before bedtime have on the body and on how you sleep, or what effect does exercise have on your body and on how you sleep? I suggest timing these things so that you maintain a regular schedule. You're going to do much better with your sleep if you have a schedule. It doesn't have to be rigid; if you go off it one night, you won't completely wreck your sleep pattern."

If exercise is part of your daily schedule (and it should be because it can increase deep sleep), it should be scheduled for late afternoon or early evening. If you're able to exercise only in the morning, it is recommended that you at least take a brisk walk in the early evening. Be wary of exercising too late in the day. Exercise performed too close to bedtime has a tendency to interfere with sleep by increasing body temperature at the time of day when it should be decreasing in anticipation of sleep. The last few hours of the day should be spent performing sedentary, relaxing activities rather than stimulating ones. "Everybody should have a wind-down time," says Posner. "If I had my way with everybody it would be four hours, but at the minimum two hours before you are planning to go to bed. This is a time when the phone calls, or at least the business calls, should be cut off. You should stop paying your bills, stop studying, stop doing work activities, and start winding down. Start doing your meditations or relaxation techniques [Section 36]; watch some TV or read."

The importance of consistency in your daily schedule cannot be overstated. Dr. Posner suggests putting a routine schedule into place and following it for about a month before deciding whether or not it improves your sleep. Don't try to determine the effectiveness of a balanced schedule in only a few days. Once you have a routine in place, stick with it for a while. You may find yourself sleeping better before the month is over.

CHAPTER THREE

KNOW YOUR SPECIAL NEEDS

#15

FOR CHILDREN ONLY: INVESTIGATE PEDIATRIC INSOMNIA

It seems that sleep and children are natural enemies—from infancy, when a baby's two A.M. cry awakens the household, to grade school when another drink and another kiss are universal bedtime-delaying tactics, to the teen years when socializing and studying rob needed sleep hours. That's why it's difficult to tell when a child truly is suffering from insomnia.

AVERAGE SLEEP NEEDS

Because sleep needs are genetically determined and generally consistent throughout one's life, your child's sleep pattern is probably not a phase—most likely it's a lifetime habit. That's why waiting for her to "grow out of it" isn't an effective solution to a sleep problem. Knowing something about the average child's sleep needs may help you evaluate your child's current sleep patterns and identify true insomnia.

According to Dr. Charles Schaefer, Ph.D., director of the

children's sleep-disorder clinic at Fairleigh Dickenson University in New Jersey and author of *Winning Bedtime Battles*, children up to two and a half years of age need ten to thirteen hours of sleep each day, three- to five-year-olds need ten to twelve hours, and six- to ten-year-olds need at least ten hours of sleep. Although these figures are only averages, it is unlikely that a child's total daily sleep time will differ by several hours. But even if it does, this doesn't automatically point to insomnia.

To evaluate your child's sleep needs and patterns, start a sleep log like the one suggested in Section 6. This will help you decide if your child is sleeping less than expected because she needs less sleep, or because she's developed poor sleep habits, or because she suffers from insomnia. Be particularly watchful of how long it takes her to fall asleep. If it generally takes a child more than thirty minutes to nod off to sleep at night, insomnia is suspect. You'll also want to stay alert to her daytime personality: On her present schedule, does she have difficulty waking in the morning? Is she regularly irritable, fatigued? Does she fall asleep in the late afternoon or early evening? Does she sleep an extra hour or more on weekends? If you answer yes to more than one of these questions, you can assume that your child needs more sleep than she is currently getting. The question now is, why?

A PROCESS OF ELIMINATION

Childhood insomnia is often diagnosed through the process of elimination. The following list of sleep zappers rule out the presence of insomnia and point to other more common causes of sleep difficulties. Consider if any of these are bothering your child:

1. *Wrong Bedtime.* Your child may lie awake for more than thirty minutes because he simply isn't tired. Try

letting him stay up later and see if he falls off to sleep with greater ease and suffers no fatigue the next day.

2. *Overstimulation.* Some persistent sleep problems happen because the child isn't physically or mentally ready for sleep. Children who go to bed still feeling stimulated from playing or watching TV may lie there for longer than a half hour waiting for the body to calm down. If your child generally jump-starts into bed, establish a calming bedtime ritual (perhaps a friendly chat, a good night story and a song) that will ease her more slowly into a sleepy frame of mind.

3. *Stress.* Like adults, children too may have trouble falling asleep when they're worried about something. The occasional stress-related sleep problem is perfectly normal and no cause for concern. But if you find that your child is continually losing sleep because he's worried about something, then it's time to investigate. Pay closer attention to his daily activities. Make time to talk over the day's events. Ask if there's anything bothering him. Listen intently to his concerns. When the root of the stress is uncovered, your child may need help learning how to relax and cope with life's ups and downs. Children can learn to use muscle massage, deep breathing, and positive self-statements to reassure themselves when their parents are sleeping and unavailable to give comfort.

4. *Poor Sleep Habits.* Many children lie awake for hours because they've developed poor sleep associations. If you sit by your daughter's bed until she falls asleep, she won't be able to get back to sleep if she wakes later in the night and you're not there. If you let your child fall asleep lying next to you while you watch TV, she won't be able to doze back off after you carry her up to bed. Many of these bad habits are started in infancy when parents rock and sing their babies to

sleep. Help your children learn to go to sleep in their beds and without your help. After a few weeks of putting themselves to sleep, their "insomnia" will be gone.

PREVENTION

It is important to prevent a normal childhood sleep problem from escalating into true insomnia. Dr. Schaefer recommends these few tips to help your children develop good sleep habits:

For Infants

- Let your baby put himself to sleep. While your child is still awake, say good night, put him down, dim the lights, and leave the room. Let him cry a few minutes just to unwind before you go in to repeat the routine.

For Preschool and School-Age Children

- If your child is having trouble sleeping at night, limit daytime naps and make them early in the day.
- Make sure your child gets plenty of exercise.
- Avoid colas, cocoa, and chocolate before bedtime. (The caffeine in one can of cola is roughly equivalent to four cups of coffee for an adult!)
- Establish a consistent bedtime so your child's internal clock is ready for sleep at night.

TRUE INSOMNIA

A relatively small number of children actually have chronic insomnia. In his book *Sleep Right in Five Nights*, Dr. James Perl notes that true childhood insomnia appears to be caused by defects in the neurological system that regulates wakefulness and sleep. Many people with childhood-onset insomnia show signs of hyperactivity or learning disabilities as children. As adults some may show unusual patterns of brain activity suggestive of neurological impairment.

If your child's sleep problem cannot be remedied with attention to the four sleep zappers explained above, true insomnia is likely the cause. Childhood insomnia is responsive to many of the suggestions outlined in this book. Read through each section carefully to gather information that will help your child establish a sleep routine that will give him the energy he needs to grow and enjoy each action-packed day of childhood.

#16

FOR TEENAGERS: WATCH FOR A SWITCH IN SLEEP PATTERNS

Seventeen-year-old Max Green goes to bed before midnight every night and gets up at six-thirty every weekday morning. On the weekends he sleeps past noon. And like most teenagers, he is always tired. "I keep telling Max to get to bed earlier on school nights," says his mom, Karen, "because he just can't wake up in the morning." Although this sounds like good advice, Max's bedtime really isn't the problem. It's his wake-up time and his weekend sleep-ins that are setting him up for problems with chronic sleep deprivation and possibly insomnia.

The nation's leading researchers in sleep disorders agree that biology may be the reason teens are chronically tired. They have observed teenagers in sleep laboratories to measure their levels of melatonin (a hormone that helps regulate the body's cycles of sleepiness and wakefulness). They have found that compared to younger children, the release of melatonin at night during the teen years signals the need for sleep later in the evening and cues wake-up time later in the morning. This makes it biologically natural to go to sleep at a later hour and rise later in the morning. Some sleep-disorder experts, like Mary A. Carskadon, a professor of psychiatry and human behavior at Brown University's School of Medicine, feel it defies nature to expect teenagers to get up early for class and perform at their peak.

Given that their school schedule is not working in sync with their body rhythms, teens try to make up for the forced lack of sleep by sleeping longer on weekends. They often sleep in until late afternoon on both Saturday and Sunday, and then Sunday night they can't fall asleep and can't get up Monday morning. This is a natural setup for sleep problems.

Because teens can't create a daily schedule that works with their body clock, they are open to sleep disorders like insomnia. Anthony Spirito, Ph.D., of the Brown University School of Medicine Sleep-Disorders Clinic, works with adolescent insomniacs. He believes that teen insomnia can be treated with many of the stimulus-control techniques (see Chapter Five) that work with adults. But because teens, more than adults, spend so much time sleeping on weekends, Dr. Spirito suggests that the first step in treating this sleep problem is to keep a bedtime and wake time that ideally stays the same all seven days of the week, at least for a few weeks. This is the hardest hurdle to get over because, being sleep-deprived, teens have a tremendous physical desire to sleep later on the weekends. But if they go to sleep at midnight and wake at six-thirty Monday through Friday, they should do the same on Saturday and Sunday. If this is too difficult, then at the very least they should get up at a reasonable hour on the weekends, like eight-thirty or nine. The body needs a consistent pattern for at least several weeks to fight off sleep disorders like insomnia that occur when sleep hours fluctuate wildly from one night to the next. Once a reasonable schedule has been reestablished, sleeping a bit later on weekends is not as likely to lead to major problems with insomnia.

#17

FOR WOMEN ESPECIALLY: KNOW HOW HORMONES AFFECT SLEEP

A nationwide survey of five hundred women, commissioned by the Better Sleep Council, turned up some unsurprising news: Women are well aware that changing hormones can incite mood swings and food cravings. Of greater interest is the fact that the survey also found that the majority of the women (56 percent) didn't know that hormones can disrupt their sleep, putting them at risk for sleep deprivation. Sleep experts know that 78 percent of the female population is in the at-risk age range for hormonal-affected sleep. This means millions of women may suffer the consequences of sleep deprivation, including daytime drowsiness, impaired concentration and judgment, and irritability. The following information about women and sleep has been gathered from a news release prepared by the Better Sleep Council called "Biological Clock Alarm: The Female Factor in Poor Sleep."

SLEEP AND HORMONES

"Men's bodies remain relatively stable throughout their lives. But women's bodies are constantly adapting to ever changing levels of hormones," says Roseanne Armitage, Ph.D., director of the Sleep Study Unit in the Psychology and Psychiatry Department at the University of Texas Southwestern Medical Center at Dallas. "The balancing act of regulating neurological and reproductive hormones is a challenge to women's systems. As a result, sleep changes during the menstrual cycle, pregnancy, and menopause."

Medical research shows that if a woman's hormones are out of kilter, her sleep will be too. Conversely, disturbed sleep patterns can cause periods to become irregular or stop altogether.

PMS AND POOR SLEEP

Drowsiness and fatigue during the menstrual cycle are the result of fluctuating levels of progesterone, a female hormone known for inducing sleep. Early in the cycle, when progesterone levels are low, women generally get less deep, restorative sleep. Mid-month ovulation triggers high levels of progesterone that makes women sleepier. With the onset of menstruation, progesterone levels plummet—setting off a night of insomnia for some women. For PMS sufferers, researchers say elevated progesterone levels may cause other changes that disrupt sleep, including increased body temperature. Research reveals that women with PMS get about one-third less deep sleep than those without symptoms. What's worse, women who suffer PMS the week prior to their periods don't get much deep sleep the entire month, making them prone to long-term sleep deprivation.

At this time there are no PMS-specific remedies for this

sleeplessness. Dr. Sharon Schutte of the Sleep Disorders Center of Thomas Jefferson University says the best way to reduce the effects of PMS on sleep is by following some of the basic insomnia-control guidelines explained throughout this book. These include: getting up about the same time every morning, taking daytime naps, and especially getting morning light exposure.

Sleep-Deprived Pregnancy

Kathryn Lee, Ph.D., associate professor of nursing at the University of California in San Francisco, asserts that pregnant women may be sleep-deprived from early pregnancy through postpartum. During pregnancy, progesterone increases daily to very high levels. While high progesterone levels usually make women sleepier, in the first trimester progesterone and its effect on other body functions—such as the increased need to urinate during the night—disrupt normal sleep patterns and thus sap daytime energy. By the twelfth week pregnant women get less of the deep sleep that restores the body, less dream-state sleep that rejuvenates the mind, and spend more time awake at night.

Through the second trimester many women seem to adapt and feel better. But in the third trimester sleep fragmentation and wakefulness increase. "The fact that pregnant women fall asleep faster is a sign of sleep deprivation—not a good sleeper," explains Lee. After delivery, infant feedings disrupt sleep, causing new mothers to run up a serious sleep deficit.

Hot Flashes and Menopause

Hot flashes are the bane of 75 percent of menopausal women—those who have them are awakened as often as every eight minutes throughout the night. That's why signs traditionally attributed to psychological problems associated with menopause like depression, fatigue, and mood swings may actually be the consequence of poor sleep.

Hot flashes are associated with reduced estrogen production and the way the body regulates temperature. Suzanne Woodward, Ph.D., assistant professor of psychiatry at Wayne State University School of Medicine in Detroit, says that estrogen therapy, which reduces the occurrence of hot flashes, can help women get a better night's sleep. But besides estrogen therapy there are no medical therapies known to stop the hot flashes and improve sleep.

Sleeping pills are not recommended for women who awake because of hot flashes. The pills may work for a night or two, but then your body needs more and more to keep up the sleep-producing effects. So in the end you're not doing yourself any good (see Chapter Four).

Dr. Woodward advises women to try to deal with this temporary sleep disturber by resting and keeping cool. You might try taking twenty-minute power naps during the day if possible. At night, try to keep your body temperature cool: wear cotton underwear that absorbs perspiration; put ice water and a fan by the bed; do some deep breathing exercises to relax; most of all try not to worry (which keeps you awake even longer). As annoying as hot flashes may be, remember that menopause is a temporary condition.

A Gallup poll conducted for the National Sleep Foundation in 1995 found that women are more likely than men to say they have sleeping difficulties (52 vs. 45 percent). This information on the effects of hormonal changes on sleep explains why. But the fact that nature may have stacked the deck of peaceful slumber against you doesn't mean you have to concede defeat. There are many controllable factors in sleep that can counter the effects of changing hormones.

Taking charge of sleep hygiene (Chapter Two), adjusting your sleep environment (Section 34), using bright-light therapy (Section 39), getting plenty of exercise (Section 37), and trying non-traditional therapies (Chapter Five) will all contribute to regaining the internal balance that fends off insomnia.

#18

For the Elderly: Learn the Difference Between Insomnia and Changing Sleep Needs

In *Moby Dick* Herman Melville wrote, "Old age is always wakeful; as if, the longer linked with life, the less man has to do with aught that looks like death." Melville was right: Insomnia is more prevalent in seniors than in any other age group. A 1990 panel of experts convened by the National Institutes of Health determined that more than half of all people sixty-five years of age and older experience disturbed sleep, and insomnia is the most common complaint. About 13 percent of the American population is sixty-five years or older. That 13 percent takes more than 30 percent of the medications prescribed by doctors (many of which affect sleep) and 40 percent of all sleeping pills. Often what is perceived as insomnia by an older sleeper is only a change in sleep length and sleep quality. It is important to distinguish between natural and/or medical changes and insomnia.

How Does Sleep Change as People Grow Older?

It's not true that the aged need less sleep than the young. But the myth persists because as individuals grow older, their bodies are less able to sustain sleep. Sleep tends to get lighter as we grow older. There seems to be more light sleep and less deep sleep with more frequent awakenings in the night, so sleep becomes more fragmented. This can be brought about by a number of things like medical conditions, the aging of the brain, less activity, and depression.

The natural change in sleep length and quality from infancy to old age is a gradual, ongoing process. Newborn infants average about 16½ hours of sleep daily until about six months of age, when the average decreases to about 14 hours. At age two the average decreases to about 12½ hours daily (including naps). At ten years of age children sleep an average of about 10 hours per day while teenagers average between 7½ to 8½ hours. During childhood about 20 to 25 percent of the night is spent in the deep delta sleep of stages three and four (see Section 1).

During adulthood significant changes in sleep occur. Time spent in Stage three and Stage four sleep (the two stages of deep sleep) is greatly reduced. In addition, nighttime awakenings become two times more likely to occur.

As individuals approach and surpass sixty years of age, they spend a mere five percent or less of the night in deep delta sleep. At age sixty, nighttime awakenings occur three times more often than at age twenty. It is clear that throughout life sleep becomes lighter and less restorative.

Also, with age the speed of your inner clock or circadian rhythm (Section 38) may have increased. Rather than running at 24 or 25 hours, it may run at 22 or 23 hours. This may be causing you to fall asleep early in the evening only to wake far too early in the morning. This type of insomnia is known as advanced sleep-phase syndrome (Section 4). Treatments for this type of insomnia are discussed later in this book.

WHICH TYPE OF SLEEP PROBLEMS ARE COMMON IN THE ELDERLY?

Because the elderly sleep more lightly, they are more susceptible to many disturbances that can affect sleep. Stimuli from both the physical environment (inside the body) and the social environment (outside the body) can disrupt a good night's sleep. With age comes changes that alter the physical environment. Discomfort from disease like arthritis, respiratory disorders, cardiovascular disorders, digestive disorders, and bladder problems can lead to nighttime disturbances. Also, conditions more common in the elderly, like sleep apnea (Section 40) and restless legs syndrome (Section 43), are likely to cause sleep problems.

Organic changes in the brain of some older people bring about an increase in agitation after dark known as sundowner's syndrome. Individuals with sundowner's syndrome need stimulation to function normally and rationally. Nighttime's decrease in stimuli and activity causes these people to become agitated, confused, and sometimes to wander off.

As mentioned before, the elderly take a large percentage of this nation's prescription medications and sleeping pills. Once in the body these drugs must be metabolized by the liver. Because the elderly often experience a decline in liver function, these drugs are metabolized at a slower rate. The result is an accumulation of the medication in the body and more notable side effects. So if a medication has a potential side effect of sleeplessness, it is more likely to appear in an elderly patient than in a younger one. Because sleeping pills are usually not metabolized quickly enough in the elderly, they can cause daytime drowsiness and hangovers that often result in falls and memory loss.

The social environment also produces many disturbances that can cause nighttime arousals. A light sleeper who sleeps with a bed partner who snores is likely to be disturbed by snoring (which had not seemed bothersome in earlier years). Elderly individuals who own pets and allow them to sleep in the same room or even in the same bed may be disturbed by the pet's nocturnal movements. Minor disturbances that were of no consequence earlier in life, such as a distant police siren or the slamming of a car door, may disrupt the light sleep of a senior. Bereavement over the loss of a loved one and physical distress like extreme room temperatures can also produce sleeplessness.

As people grow older, they are more likely to spend time in unfamiliar surroundings such as their children's homes, hospitals, nursing homes, sheltered housing, or residential homes for the elderly. Laboratory experiments have proven that unfamiliar surroundings and a change in daily schedule can lead to sleep problems.

How Can You Improve Your Sleep?

As you grow older, it is important that you remain active mentally, socially, and physically. A 1988 Gallup survey indicated that active retirees registered fewer sleep complaints than those who were less active. When people exercise, it tends to increase the depth of their sleep.

Nevertheless, recent research indicates that the body is designed for at least one afternoon nap per day. With few daily commitments, retirees are often able to take advantage of nature's calling. If you decide to nap during the day, however, be aware that napping will reduce your nighttime sleep by roughly the duration of the nap.

On nights when you go to bed and find it impossible to fall asleep, Dr. Michael Stevenson, clinical director of North Valley Sleep Disorders Center, Mission Hills, California, suggests that you practice a form of stimulus control. If you wake in the middle of the night, lie in your bed with your eyes wide open while concentrating on your breathing. "This quickly lets you know if you are sleepy or not because it is very hard to hold your eyes open if you're sleepy," he says. If you are not sleepy, get out of bed. Once out of bed, perform a sedentary activity like reading, watching television, or working on a quiet hobby until you can no longer hold your eyes open. Then get back into bed and let yourself fall asleep.

"You should give yourself about a half hour to fall asleep before getting out of bed," says Stevenson. "But don't become a clock watcher. Watching the clock may raise your anxiety level, making it that much more difficult to fall asleep."

Following the advice in this section, combined with good medical care, a proper diet, and daily exercise, may help you get a deeper, more restorative, and higher-quality night's sleep.

CHAPTER FOUR

THINK TWICE ABOUT SLEEPING PILLS

#19

EXPLORE HOW SLEEPING PILLS WORK

Sleeping pill is a very broad term that is used to refer to any chemical agent that affects the central nervous system and produces drowsiness. This includes antihistamines, barbiturates, antidepressants, benzodiazepines, and nonbenzodiazepine medications. When used to bring on sleep, these drugs are all called hypnotics. (The sleep induced by hypnotic drugs does not resemble the state of suggestibility brought on through hypnosis.)

Although all hypnotics are supposed to promote sleep, each has a unique influence on several aspects of sleep and well-being. They may affect what researchers and sleep specialists call sleep latency—the time between lying down in bed and actually falling asleep. They may work to increase sleep duration—the length of time you stay asleep without waking. They also may affect the quality of your sleep, influence your dreams and have an effect on your ability to function the following day.

Sleep medications can differ in the way they influence

your sleep, but they all work by depressing the central nervous system—a process causing reactions that include anxiety, suppression of inhibitions, sedation, and sleep.

NOT REALLY SLEEP

Thirty-eight-year-old Steven McKay had just returned home from a twelve-day business trip to Tokyo. It was midnight at home, but he was wide awake and suffering from jet lag. "When that happens," he says, "I take a sleeping pill so I can get a good night's sleep before I go back to the office the next day."

Hypnotic drugs do bring on sleep, but they don't give you what can be called "good" sleep. There are clear-cut differences between drug-induced and non-drug sleep. Researchers report that all hypnotic medications distort the normal sleep patterns by altering the time spent in the various sleep stages. (See Section 1 for a full discussion of sleep stages.) It has not been established that interfering with any sleep stage is detrimental, but many sleep specialists find it disturbing that hypnotic medications produce regular and long-term changes involving portions of sleep considered most important. REM sleep (which is often reduced in drug-induced sleep) is believed to play an important role in maintaining the balance of functions and chemical composition within the brain as well as in learning and memory consolidation. Stages three and four, which are drastically reduced by hypnotics called benzodiazepines, are the portions of sleep thought to be important in terms of protein synthesis and tissue repair. So those who think nothing of popping a little pill to get a "good night's sleep" may actually be interfering with vital functions assigned to the brain during sleep hours.

Not only do sleeping pills impair the function of sleep, they also affect the way you feel the next day. Because sleep medication often reduces stages three and four (deep sleep), the night's sleep is less refreshing than natural sleep. And because sleeping pills increase shallow sleep in stages one and two, they can cause more periods of wakefulness during the night; this too will leave you feeling less refreshed in the morning.

The more you learn about sleeping pills (the good and the bad), the more you'll understand why, used alone, they are not a recommended therapy for the treatment of insomnia.

But what is best, taking a pill, or not sleeping et all?

20

WATCH OUT FOR
SIDE EFFECTS

Anyone taking sleeping pills should know that there are negative side effects that accompany their use. Many of these are specific to individual drugs and are explained in sections 22 and 23, but the following general precautions apply to all hypnotics.

1. Sleeping pills act on the central nervous system. This can reduce the functioning capacity of such basic processes as breathing and vision, and lessen alertness and natural reflexes.
2. Some sleep medications accumulate in the body and cause a hangover feeling the next day.
3. Certain medical conditions increase the risk of taking sleeping pills. For instance, in patients with sleep apnea or asthma when respiratory function is borderline, the additional respiratory depression caused by any sleeping pill can be life-threatening. Also, anyone with serious liver or kidney disease may not metab-

olize or excrete medication properly and so may be in danger from much smaller doses of sleeping pills than most people.

4. Sleeping pills can interfere with the effect of other medications and can be dangerous when combined with them. Be sure to tell your physician about all other medications, both prescription and over-the-counter, that you take at any time. Also, watch your intake of alcohol and illicit drugs like marijuana. Taking sleeping pills and other depressants can kill you.

THE CYCLE OF ABUSE

"I don't get it," complained night-shift nurse Maura Stevenson to the doctor on duty. "Last week I started taking these sleeping pills to help me get some sleep during the day while the kids are at school, and they worked great—I slept long and sound and woke up feeling great. But this week I take them and nothing happens; I can't sleep. Should I double the dosage?"

The doctor explained to Maura that doubling the dosage is a bad idea that will only compound her sleep problems. Sleeping pills work effectively for only a short period of time; they cannot maintain their effectiveness for weeks on end (and certainly not months or years!). This fact causes many insomniacs to get caught up in a cycle of drug abuse that requires higher and higher dosages and finally causes physical and/or psychological dependence. Beware of signs of the following trouble.

Tolerance

Tolerance develops when the effect of the original dose of the sleeping pill diminishes, leading the user to need more and more of the drug to achieve the same response. Most hypnotics appear to lose their sleep-promoting properties within three to fourteen days of continuous use. The natural inclination is to increase the dosage to continue the benefits. But when the highest allowable dosage is achieved, it's a dead-end situation. When the body develops tolerance to a prescribed pill, some people ask their physicians to give them a different pill. This is not effective, however, because in most cases, if you are tolerant to one kind of drug, a benzodiazepine for example, you will have developed tolerance to the other drugs in that family as well.

Rebound

A serious problem with the use of hypnotics, particularly shorter-acting ones, is rebound insomnia. This occurs when pills are discontinued and the symptoms of insomnia become much worse than they were before taking the medication. For example, as much as a 60 percent increase in total awake time has been reported on the first night following discontinuation of the drug triazolam. Anxiety, which may have been eased by the hypnotic treatment, may also rebound. Although rebound is a temporary reaction, it tends to reinforce insomniacs' belief that they cannot sleep without medication. This pushes them to return to medication and sets the stage for dependency.

Dependence

Very gradually, and often without notice, people who use sleeping pills find that they need the pill to maintain a sense of physical or psychological ease. Even though the medication may have lost its initial beneficial effects, they believe they cannot stop taking the pill.

Withdrawal

When sleeping pills are discontinued after long-term treatment (particularly longer-acting hypnotics), many people suffer withdrawal symptoms. These include general malaise, vision problems, and increases in anxiety and insomnia. In some patients depression becomes quite severe.

Obviously, sleeping pills are not harmless; they are drugs that require caution and care in use. The next section will give you an idea of when sleeping pills are and are not an appropriate remedy for insomnia.

#21

KNOW WHO CAN AND WHO CANNOT USE SLEEPING PILLS

In general, drug therapy is effective only for a very short period and even then only when used with other behavioral therapies and/or psychological counseling.

In a few circumstances, however, it is sometimes appropriate to use a sleeping pill:

1. If you are under unusual stress that already has caused you to lose a night or more of sleep, sleeping pills for *only* a night or two might put your sleep back on track.
2. If you suffer from periodic insomnia and have tried without relief non-drug treatments such as the relaxation response, sleeping pills may be useful. However, you should continue to explore the causes of your insomnia and other methods of treatment.
3. You may experience sleep difficulties caused by pain associated with surgery or other medical conditions such as arthritis. In these cases sleep problems can sometimes be temporarily treated with sleeping pills.

4. There are rare cases in which no underlying cause can be found for a person's insomnia. These cases are sometimes treated with sleeping pills under the careful supervision of a physician.

Short-term use of a hypnotic may be all that is required to promote a normal sleep habit. During this time it's important to follow prescribing directions for when and how much to take, to resist increasing the amount, and to take them for no longer than a few weeks unless directed by a physician.

Once the transient sleep problem has passed, stop taking the sleeping pills. People who continue using the pills "just in case I can't sleep" end up dependent on the pill and subject to the problems outlined in the previous section.

Even for short-term, temporary relief of insomnia, you should not take any kind of sleeping pill if you:

- are pregnant
- are a nursing mother
- have had any alcohol
- are taking certain other medications (ask your doctor)
- need to be alert during the night (for example, if you are on call for work emergencies) or early the next morning
- have liver or kidney disease

The use of hypnotic drugs in the treatment of long-term insomnia is controversial, not only because of the likelihood of tolerance and potential drug abuse, but also because this condition is often secondary to disorders that are manageable by psychotherapy, physical therapy, chronotherapy, or non-hypnotic drugs. Sleeping specialists believe that long-term use of sleeping pills should be restricted to a fairly small group of patients. This group includes those who have severe insomnia for which no clear medical or psychiatric cause has been established, or when a cause has been established but no adequate or specific treatment has been found. But even in this group only a small number will benefit because hypnotics often lose their effectiveness with time. Long-term use should also be avoided because there is evidence suggesting that chronic use of hypnotics exacerbates rather than relieves the difficulties of an insomniac.

#22

THINK AGAIN ABOUT
OVER-THE-COUNTER
SLEEPING PILLS

Mark Tyreak, a college student, was dead tired. Usually after going to classes and working his part-time job, Mark fell asleep quickly when he finally crawled into bed at night. But for the past four nights he had tossed and turned, unable to sleep at all. "Maybe I'll go to the pharmacy and buy some sleeping pills," he told his roommate. "I'll use them just until exams are over. What harm can it do?"

Mark can easily get over-the-counter (OTC) drugs—those you can buy without a prescription. Popular OTC sleeping pills include Sominex, Nytol, and Compoze. These and other OTCs contain antihistamines that, along with their effect on a stuffy nose, can make you feel drowsy.

Although OTC products can be purchased without a prescription, that doesn't mean they are harmless. Like prescription drugs, they affect the central nervous system and should be used with caution and not be used more than a few nights in a row.

The primary side effect of OTC sleeping aids is the occurrence of a mental slowdown; they can make it difficult to concentrate, focus, or drive a car. Other reactions to antihistamines include:

- ringing in the ears
- dizziness
- blurred vision
- loss of appetite
- nausea or vomiting

OTC sleeping pills are usually ineffective for all but the milder, temporary forms of insomnia. Since they work quickly but don't last very long, these products work only to help you fall asleep. They can't help with frequent nighttime awakenings.

23

INVESTIGATE PRESCRIPTION MEDICATIONS

Although prescription sleeping pills are lumped together under the umbrella term *hypnotics*, each is quite different from the other in its formulation, action, use, and potential for side effects. If you are taking prescription sleeping pills or have considered using them to treat your insomnia, you need to find out more about them. Then you'll know why drug therapy alone is not a cure for insomnia.

THE NAME GAME

To fully understand sleep medication, you'll need to play the name game to decipher the four different labels carried by each drug. Let's look at the drug triazolam as an example:

- This drug is sold under the brand name *Halcion*, which is the label used by the pharmaceutical manufacturer to market the drug.

- *Triazolam* is the chemical or generic name for Halcion.
- *Benzodiazepine* is the chemical family to which triazolam belongs.
- Because triazolam is often prescribed to induce sleep, it belongs to the group of drugs called *hypnotics*.

If your doctor prescribes a hypnotic, ask which one. If she says it's a benzodiazepine, ask which one. If she gives you the brand name, ask for the generic name as well. This information gives you what you need to do some research of your own.

WHAT YOU NEED TO KNOW

Taking a sleeping pill seems easy enough: Insert in mouth and swallow. But once the pill is absorbed into your bloodstream, there's a lot more going on that you should know about. You need to know:

- who should and should not take this medication
- which side effects (like dizziness, dry mouth, diarrhea, etc.) are associated with this medication
- which adverse reactions can occur, signaling you to immediately stop taking the drug
- which other medications or activities should be avoided while taking the drug
- which medical conditions rule out the use of this drug

The answers to these questions can be found easily in any local library. There are many books that describe prescription and non-prescription drugs. A most popular source of information is the *Physicians Desk Reference*, which helps you identify your medication by showing color pictures and then giving the details of its use.

CLASSES OF DRUGS

Several classes of prescribed medications are commonly used in the treatment of insomnia: barbiturates, antidepressants, benzodiazepines, and nonbenzodiazepine hypnotics. Take a look at what these "sleeping pills" do to promote sleep.

Barbiturates

Barbiturates are a major class of hypnotics that have been in use since the early 1900s. The barbiturates used primarily as hypnotics are pentobarbital (Nembutal), secobarbital (Seconal), and amobarbital (Amytal).

Once the first line of treatment for insomnia, barbiturates have now been almost completely abandoned for this use. They have a higher level of toxicity than other available hypnotics, they are more likely to interact negatively with other medications, and they pose a greater risk for developing tolerance and dependence. Also, an overdose of barbiturates can severely depress the central nervous system and lead to death.

Barbiturates are no longer a recommended form of drug therapy for insomnia.

Antidepressants

Antidepressants with sedative effects are usually recommended when insomnia is associated with a depressive disorder. These include doxepin (Adapin, Sinequan), trazodone (Desyrel), trimipramine (Surmontil), and amitriptyline (Elavil). Many physicians prescribe antidepressants rather than benzodiazepines for treating insomnia even in nondepressed patients because the potential for abuse or physical dependency is lower. But because the potential for drug interactions is higher than with benzodiazepines, they are not recommended for people who are taking other medications.

Benzodiazepines

Benzodiazepines are much safer than the older barbiturates and are said to be a popular choice among physicians for treating insomnia. Although there are many benzodiazepines on the market, only five are approved for the treatment of insomnia: flurazepam (Dalmane), temazepam (Restoril), triazolam (Halcion), quazepam (Doral), and estazolam (ProSom). Selection of the appropriate drug depends on the kind of insomnia a patient has. For example, if a patient needs medication to accelerate falling asleep, a benzodiazepine with a rapid onset of action (like triazolam) would be prescribed. However, if medication is needed to prevent waking later in the night, a benzodiazepine with a slower onset (like estazolam) is needed.

All these drugs are most effectively used for transient or short-term insomnia, for which prescriptions should, if possible, be limited to a few days, occasional or intermittent use, or courses not exceeding two weeks.

All benzodiazepines promote sleep in one or all of the following ways: (1) they reduce the amount of time needed to fall asleep; (2) they decrease the number and duration of nighttime awakenings; and (3) they increase total sleep time. Benzodiazepines differ in how quickly they affect sleep and how long effects last.

Although benzodiazepines have a reputation for causing only a low incidence of abuse and dependence, the possibility of adverse side effects does exist. *The Pharmacological Basis of Therapeutics* by Goodman and Gilman states that at the time of peak concentration, benzodiazepines can be expected to cause varying degrees of lightheadedness, fatigue, slower reaction time, motor and neurological incoordination, impairment of mental and psychomotor functions, disorganization of thought, and confusion. All of these effects greatly impair driving and psychomotor skills. For example, in one study the residual effects of two nightly 30-mg doses of flurazepam on driving performance were at least as great as those produced acutely by alcohol at a concentration of 100 mg/dl in blood, a level at which persons usually are considered legally intoxicated.

Other relatively common side effects of benzodiazepines are weakness, headache, blurred vision, vertigo, nausea and vomiting, diarrhea, joint pains, and chest pains. With long-term use dependence and withdrawal effects can become major disadvantages. They also increase stage two sleep, and decrease the amount of stages three and four sleep, which is considered the most restorative sleep.

Patients rarely develop tolerance to benzodiazepines used as hypnotics. However, anyone tolerant to barbiturates, alcohol, and other general central nervous system depressants show some cross-tolerance to benzodiazepines.

Physiological dependence on benzodiazepines can occur and is accompanied by a withdrawal syndrome. Withdrawal from normal dosage benzodiazepine treatment can result in a number of symptomatic patterns. The most common is a short-lived "rebound" anxiety and insomnia, coming within one to four days of discontinuation. The second pattern is the full-blown withdrawal syndrome, usually lasting one to eleven days; finally, a third pattern may represent the return of anxiety symptoms that then persist until some form of treatment is instituted.

Withdrawal symptoms appear to be more severe following withdrawal from high doses or from short-acting benzodiazepines. This is typically characterized by sleep disturbance, irritability, increased tension and anxiety, panic attacks, hand tremors, sweating, difficulty in concentration, dry retching and nausea, some weight loss, palpitations, headache, muscular pain and stiffness and a host of vision problems.

In spite of the adverse effects, the benzodiazepines are relatively safe drugs. Even huge doses are rarely fatal unless taken along with other drugs.

Zolpidem

Zolpidem (Ambien) is a nonbenzodiazepine hypnotic. It has a rapid onset of action and is useful in both initiating and maintaining sleep. It seems to have a minimal effect on sleep stages and therefore is thought to promote a more natural sleep. It is recommended for the short-term management of insomnia. Typically, prescriptions for this drug provide a maximum of one month's supply.

Zolpidem has several advantages over benzodiazepines: lack of withdrawal effects, reduced likelihood of rebound insomnia, and little or no tolerance.

According to *Pharmacology for Nursing Care*, the possible side effects of zolpidem are similar to those of the benzodiazepines. Daytime drowsiness and dizziness are most common, and these occur in only one to two percent of patients. The likelihood of these types of side effects increases as the dose of the drug is increased. No impairment of performance is evident during the day after its use. However, if a patient wakens during the night when the drug effect is still present, impaired short-term memory, psychomotor performance, and unsteady gait may occur. Short-term treatment is not associated with significant tolerance or physical dependence. Withdrawal symptoms are minimal or absent.

Zolpidem should not be used by patients with sleep apnea, since it worsens the apnea.

#24

KNOW HOW SLEEPING PILLS
AFFECT THE ELDERLY

Seventy-year-old Jake Williams was slowing down. He felt
unusually tired during the day. He started dozing off while
watching TV. He had trouble driving without his eyelids feeling heavy. "What's going on?" he asked his doctor. "You gave
me sleeping pills so I could sleep better at night, but I think
they're making me feel sleepy all day long. Is that possible?"

It is not only possible but common for sleeping pills to
noticeably affect the daytime functioning of the elderly.
Physiological changes that normally accompany the aging
process alter absorption, distribution, excretion, and drug metabolism. That's why older adults are more sensitive to drugs
and their side effects than younger people.

Long-acting drugs, like many sleeping pills, are especially detrimental to the elderly. They can create nocturnal
confusion, can result in cognitive and motor impairment, and
can increase the risks of falls. In a study called "Falls among
the Institutionalized Elderly," Perlin and associates reported
that at the time of the falls, 60 patients (81 percent) were

taking drugs that affect the central nervous system. Daytime carryover effects, such as sleepiness and reduced alertness, are also more pronounced in the medicated elderly.

The side effects of sleeping pills are compounded in the elderly by the increased possibility for multiple-drug interactions. Elderly patients are very likely to be using medication for other conditions such as diabetes, heart disease, hypertension, or arthritis. These medications may influence the way a sleeping pill works. Conversely, a sleeping pill may alter the expected effect of the other medications. Americans over age sixty-five take more than 30 percent of the medications prescribed by doctors, and 40 percent of all sleeping pills. These numbers say that there are bound to be negative interactions in the drug-sensitive elderly.

Even OTC sleeping aids are not a good choice for older people. OTC antihistamines have an effect on the production of the compound released at the autonomic nerve endings that are active in the transmission of the nerve impulse. Also, they generally do not include special usage and dosage instructions for the elderly and can put an older person at risk for delirium.

Because the elderly react to sleeping pills differently from the younger population and because it's likely they take other pills along with sleeping pills, it is especially important for the elderly to monitor their use of sleep medications. Your physician must know about *all* other medications you are taking. You need to try behavioral therapies that promote sleep (like relaxation, diet, and schedule changes) and consider giving up sleeping pills. As the next section points out, sleeping pills never cure insomnia.

It's most important to remember when evaluating the benefits of sleeping pills that insomnia is not an illness in itself, but rather a symptom of a number of different underlying conditions. Among these are depression, anxiety, numerous medical diseases, pain, environmental conditions, and the side effects of medications.

A sleeping pill masks the cause by covering up the symptom, but it doesn't get rid of the problem. If you really want to cure yourself of nightly battles with insomnia, you must identify the factors that are causing your insomnia and deal with them. That's the only effective long-term solution. Reliance on sleeping pills sentences you to a life of sleeplessness and ultimately addiction to pills that no longer work.

25

LOOK AT WHAT'S NEW

Up to now insomniacs have relied on medications that depress the central nervous system, and have suffered the side effects and dangers of this route to sound sleep. Now a new medication based on the naturally occurring hormone melatonin is making headlines and offering hope of a nonaddictive form of sleeping pill.

Melatonin is a hormone found naturally in the pineal gland, a tiny timekeeper in the brain that sets the body's clock to the cycles of night and day. When the sun goes down, the eyes cue the gland to start pumping melatonin. In response, body temperature falls, metabolism slows, and we prepare to drop off. As the morning light appears, the gland reduces its output, allowing the body to gradually come back to life. The gland functions this way throughout our lives, although it secretes less and less melatonin with age (that may be one reason why so many elderly people have trouble sleeping).

A synthetic form of melatonin can be bought over-the-counter at health food stores and many pharmacies. This alternative drug has received an open-armed welcome from insomniacs around the world. The appearance of a drug that promotes sleep without depressing the central nervous system has been long awaited.

Many studies have been conducted to test the effectiveness of melatonin on sleep. Richard J. Wurtman, Ph.D., of the Massachusetts Institute of Technology, reported that melatonin functioned naturally as a sleep-inducing hormone even in very small doses. His volunteers fell asleep in five to six minutes on melatonin, while those on a placebo took about fifteen minutes longer.

In the Technion Medical School in Haifa, Israel, Peretz Lavie, M.D., and associates found similar results. Their study found that nine men and women ages sixty-eight to eighty who took melatonin had less trouble falling asleep and slept longer without waking up. The time required to fall asleep on melatonin was cut from forty to fifteen minutes, and the volunteers said that they had a more refreshing sleep.

Nava Zisapel of Tel Aviv University says, "The major effect we found with melatonin was in sleep maintenance. People could fall back asleep much more easily after waking in the middle of the night." In Zisapel's study the volunteers fell asleep more quickly and slept about 10 percent longer when taking the melatonin than while taking the placebo.

Writing in *Natural Prescriptions*, Robert M. Giller, M.D., advises taking a 2 mg capsule each night for two weeks; if you notice no results, then you should discontinue its use.

So far melatonin appears to be safe, at least for short-term use. But there is some concern that melatonin may affect the female reproductive system. Doctors have shown that daily melatonin doses of around 250 mg suppress ovulation when used with other hormones. Dutch researchers are now testing it as a contraceptive. "The long-term effect of melatonin on women is totally unexplored territory right now," says David Oren of the National Institute of Mental Health. "Any woman who experiments with the hormone should know that."

There is lots of speculation, both scientific and financial, about the future of melatonin in the treatment of insomnia. Pharmaceutical giants like Glaxo Wellcome and Eli Lilly are now testing melatonin as a sleeping aid. It would not be surprising to see melatonin soon become a prescription item.

CHAPTER FIVE

CHECK OUT NON-TRADITIONAL THERAPIES

#26

Shop for Foods That Encourage Peaceful Sleep

It is common knowledge that a well-balanced diet promotes good health. Nutrients provide the body with calories (the raw building materials needed for growth and maintenance) and with substances that aid regulation of body processes. But few people know that diet can also be an effective weapon in the battle against insomnia. According to Brian Clement, director of the Hippocrates Health Institute in West Palm Beach, Florida, the major nutrients related to sleep are minerals and trace minerals. If you routinely deprive your body of these minerals, your diet may be contributing to your insomnia.

Inorganic Nutrients

Minerals are inorganic nutrients and are broken into two categories: macronutrients (minerals the body needs in fairly large amounts) and micronutrients, or trace elements (needed in tiny amounts). A lot of mineralization is needed to create a sedative effect, calm the nerves and promote sound sleep.

Macronutrients That Promote Sleep

Calcium. The macronutrient calcium is known to have a calming effect on the central nervous system. Although calcium is essential for human life, most Americans do not get adequate amounts of this mineral. There are several reasons for this deficiency. The first is diet. Because calcium is found in foods that are high in fat and cholesterol (milk, cheese, and eggs), many people who are watching their weight and cholesterol intake have eliminated these foods from their diets, thus limiting their calcium intake.

The second reason for calcium deficiency is the fact that the body has difficulty absorbing the mineral. Although calcium may be present in many foods, other substances like oxalic acid (found in spinach) and phytic acid (found in the bran of whole grains) bind up the calcium, preventing its absorption.

Excess protein in the diet and daily stress also contribute to calcium deficiency. Protein and stress produce high concentrations of lactic acid in the blood; to neutralize the acidity, the bones release significant amounts of calcium and phosphorous, causing a depletion of these minerals. (At age fifty the body's ability to absorb calcium may diminish, further aggravating this situation.)

The National Research Council suggests the following daily intake of calcium:

- 1,200 milligrams for males and females ages eleven to twenty-four
- 800 milligrams after age twenty-four
- 1,200 milligrams for pregnant women and nursing mothers

Some researchers suggest 1,500 milligrams daily for post-menopausal women and 1,000 milligrams daily for premeno-pausal women.

Foods rich in calcium are: milk, cheese, ice cream, eggs, yogurt, buttermilk, salmon, broccoli, cauliflower, green leafy vegetables, figs, oranges, almonds, soy beans, and turnip greens.

Magnesium. Magnesium is a macronutrient and a natural sedative. It also aids the body's ability to absorb calcium. If a diet includes the recommended daily allowances of calcium but does not include the recommended daily allowance of magnesium, the calcium will not be fully absorbed by the body.

The National Research Council recommends:

- 350 milligrams daily for men
- 280 milligrams daily for women
- 320 milligrams daily for pregnant women
- 340 to 355 milligrams daily for nursing mothers

Foods rich in magnesium are: meats, seafood, green vegetables, and dairy products.

Micronutrients That Promote Sleep

Trace amounts of copper, iron, zinc, and aluminum play some role in limiting the occurrence of insomnia. Researchers at the U.S. Department of Agriculture research center in Grand Forks, North Dakota, found that a deficiency in iron and copper, and an overabundance of aluminum (as found in antacids), caused some women to have sleep problems. Rich sources of copper are liver, oysters, chickpeas, Brazil nuts, and cashews. Rich sources of iron include meat, fish, poultry, beets, dried beans, leafy green vegetables, and sea vegetables.

As a group, sea vegetables such as dulse and kelp are one of the richest food sources of minerals and trace elements. They can be eaten as snacks, they are pleasant additions to soups, or they can be purchased in powder form as a healthy and tasty salt replacement.

ORGANIC NUTRIENTS

In addition to inorganic nutrients, your body needs organic nutrients. Some that have been found to be useful in combating insomnia include the following.

Vitamin B$_3$ (niacin) is sometimes used to relieve insomnia caused by mild depression. Studies conducted by Dr. Connie Robinson of the University of Alabama Department of Neurosciences have shown that niacin prolonged REM sleep and decreased the time spent awake by insomniacs. B$_3$ has also helped insomniacs who fall asleep quickly but have problems remaining asleep.

The National Research Council recommends 13 to 19 milligrams of niacin daily for adults. Infants should get 5 to 6 milligrams, and children ages 1 to 10 should get 9 to 13 milligrams daily.

Niacin can be found in peanuts, sunflower seeds, red hot peppers, tomatoes, kelp sea vegetable, lean meats, poultry, and fish.

Vitamin B$_6$ (pyridoxine) acts as a natural sedative on the nerves and is instrumental in maintaining the proper level of magnesium in the blood. When B$_6$ is deficient, the amino acid tryptophan is not used properly by the body. (You'll learn more about tryptophan later in this chapter.)

The Food and Drug Administration recommends two

milligrams of B_6 each day for adults. Foods that contain B_6 are meats (particularly organ meats), whole grains, brewer's yeast, bananas, and potatoes.

B_{12} is another B vitamin that has been used to treat insomnia. Drs. Behrooz Kamgar-Parsi, Thomas Wehr, and J. Christian Gillin of the National Institute of Mental Health reported in the journal *Sleep* in 1983 that they were able to maintain normal sleep-wake cycles in a patient who had been an insomniac for ten years simply by administering B_{12} supplements.

B_{12} is found in bean sprouts, dulse sea vegetable, fish, dairy products, organ meats, eggs, beef, and pork. The recommended daily allowance of B_{12} is three milligrams daily.

Note that B complex vitamins are depleted by nicotine, alcohol, stress, and oral contraceptives.

WHAT ELSE SHOULD I LOOK FOR?

Tryptophan is a naturally occurring amino acid. Inside the body tryptophan is carried to the brain, where it is converted into the neurotransmitter chemical serotonin; serotonin induces sleep. Research indicates that about 50 percent of insomniacs are helped by dietary increases of tryptophan. (In 1989 a synthetic form of tryptophan was taken off the market because of side effects due to contaminants used in the manufacturing of the drug.)

To increase your intake of this amino acid, increase your intake of these foods: milk, meats, fish, poultry, eggs, beans, peanuts, cheese, and leafy green vegetables.

Carbohydrates may be another source of sound sleep for you. Dr. Stevens recommends that insomniacs eat a complex-carbohydrate snack (such as crackers, cereal, bread, or pasta) before bed. This tends to increase sleep maintenance, letting you sleep more deeply and reducing the likelihood that you'll wake during the night.

LOOKING IN ALL THE WRONG PLACES

Thirty-two-year-old Kara Miller is quite typical of many insomniacs. Kara grabs a doughnut for breakfast, a quick sandwich for lunch, and a burger for dinner, and some chips or cookies before heading to bed. "I'm not under a lot of stress," she says, "and I don't drink a lot of coffee. Why can't I fall asleep at night?"

The root of Kara's problem could lie in a nutritional deficiency. What you eat or don't eat can play a role in your insomnia. You may want to shop for the foods listed in this section and be sure to get the recommended daily allowances of the vitamins and minerals. Eating a well-balanced diet may not only alleviate your insomnia, it may improve your overall health.

#27

TRY HERBAL REMEDIES

As far back as 400 B.C., Hippocrates, the father of medicine, was using diet to cure his patients' ills. He viewed herbs as a virtual cure-all. Although many ailments cannot be cured by herbs, people have found that their stress-related insomnia is relieved when herbs are introduced. Brian Clement, a nutritionist and director of the Hippocrates Health Institute in Florida, uses an herbal product that is a powerful sedative. "It's called Lights Out," Clement says, "and it's a combination of herbs that effectively takes the blood chemistry and changes it as it goes into the brain."

HOW DO HERBS WORK?

Some herbs have a tranquilizing effect on the human body. Tiny alkaloids from the herbs saturate the blood and are carried to the brain. Inside the brain these alkaloids act as a circulatory sedative by "clicking off" parts of the brain.

WHICH HERBS ARE MOST EFFECTIVE
FOR INSOMNIACS?

Here is a look at four herbs that exhibit sedative properties.

Valerian Root. Valerian root has been used for centuries as a mild sedative. Before barbiturates were invented in the early 1900s, valerian root was the most widely used sedative. In World War I it was used by troops on the front lines to prevent shell shock, and in World War II it was used by civilians experiencing stress and anxiety from air raids. Valerian root is most often used to treat sleep disorders that stem from anxiety and nervousness.

Hops. Hops are usually combined with other herbs (such as valerian root and passion flower) to calm nerves and induce sleep. A combination of hops, passion flower, valerian root, and melissa is used to form Vita-Dor, a sleeping aid marketed in Germany. Hops have also been stuffed into pillows, taking the place of down to help induce sleep. In high amounts hops are such a potent sedative that Clement, working as an herbalist, offers them to dental patients.

Passion Flower. Passion flower was discovered in Peru by a Spanish doctor named Monardes in 1569. The herb became very popular in Europe, where it was used to brew tea. Passion flower is employed around the world as a mild sedative that reduces nervous tension and anxiety. In Europe and Russia passion flower is coupled with valerian root to create some very popular sleeping aids. Passion flower is also effective in combating muscle cramps that disrupt and limit sleep.

Chamomile. Chamomile (sometimes spelled *camomile*) is the most frequently used of the sleep-inducing herbs. Both chamomile tea and chamomile preparations are used for the depressive effect they have on the central nervous system. "If you took chamomile and extracted it and put in a tincture [alcohol solution] and you had just the medicinal part of the plant, you would have a very strong sedative," says Clement. Also, because chamomile has the ability to act as a carminative (expels the gas from the stomach or bowel), it may be effective to those who lose sleep due to indigestion or gas pains.

Lavender. A study out of the University of Leicester in England and published in the British medical journal *Lancet* reported that the sweet smell of lavender oil helped four elderly insomniacs fall asleep more quickly and sleep longer. Three of them stopped taking sedatives. "The results are very intriguing and very consistent with what we and others have found," says Dr. Alan Hirsch, director of the Smell and Taste Research Center in Chicago. Hirsch says the olfactory bulb, the nose's nerve center, lies close to the brain's reticular activating system, which controls the sleep-wake cycle. He speculates that chemicals in the lavender oil flow through the nose into the brain, somehow altering the biology of the sleep center.

Where Can I Get Herbs?

A health food store is a good place to search for the herbs listed above. They are sold in three forms: extract, capsule, and loose. The extract from an herb can be either brewed in a tea or taken directly into the mouth. If the flavor of an herb you have chosen is undesirable, you may want to buy your herbs in capsule form. Capsules can be swallowed or dissolved in water to form a nostrum. If you prefer to take capsules and would like to save some money, you can buy loose herbs, empty capsules, and a device that helps you fill the capsules. If you decide to brew a tea with a combination of herbs, you can purchase the herbs in loose or bulk form. If this is the route you choose, you will need to invest in either an infuser (stainless steel ball that allows you to steep the herbs in water) or sachet bags (reusable cloth tea bags).

Products such as Nighty Night and Celestial Seasonings Sleepytime save you the trouble of buying the herbs and brewing a combination. These products have most of the herbs discussed here already combined into tea bags ready to be steeped. These can be purchased at health food stores or supermarkets.

Several books have been written on the subject of herbs and herbal remedies. The following discuss the use and effects of the herbs mentioned, plus many more in greater detail: *Medical Botany* by W. J. Simmonite, *Back to Eden: An Herbal Guide* by Jethro Kloss, and *Herbal Tonic Remedies* by Daniel B. Mowrey.

WARNING: If you decide to mix herbs, whether in teas or in capsules, please consult your doctor or sleep specialist first. Although the herbs mentioned are harmless to most people, allergic reactions can occur.

28

LOOK INTO
HOMEOPATHIC TREATMENTS

Homeopathy is a system of health care and treatment that was developed in the 1800s by Dr. Samuel Hahnemann. The philosophy of homeopathy is based on the holistic idea that the mental and physical realms are inseparable. Hahnemann believed that orthodox medicine was a system of "contraries," meaning that doctors treated the symptoms of an illness by using drugs that oppose, or suppress, them. He began to call conventional medicine *allopathic*, meaning "different" and "disease, suffering." Hahnemann recognized that removing or masking symptoms did not treat the underlying cause of the illness, which could, in effect, develop into a more serious condition.

In homeopathy symptoms are seen as a healthy response of the body's defense mechanism. When the body is threatened by some harmful external influence, the defense mechanisms produce symptoms in its struggle against the harmful agent. Therefore, to a homeopathic doctor fever is a sign that the body is fighting illness. A cough (which an allopathic doctor would try to suppress with medication) is seen by the homeopath as the natural way to expel mucus from the body. The homeopathic treatment is one that produces the same symptoms that the person is complaining of, and in doing so sharply provokes the body into throwing them off.

Hahnemann discovered that certain remedies caused particular symptoms in a healthy person. But when that remedy was given to a sick person exhibiting those same symptoms, it helped cure the person. Based on this notion that like cures like, Hahnemann formulated the Law of Similars. It states that a substance causing certain symptoms in a healthy person can cure a sick person with the same symptoms. The theory behind the Law of Similars is that the body enlists its own energies to heal itself and defend against illness. If a substance that causes a similar response in terms of similar symptoms is administered, the body steps up its fight against it, thereby promoting a cure. Thus the name *homeopathy*, which comes from the Greek words *omio* (meaning "same") and *pathos* (meaning "suffering").

Based on Hippocrates' order "first, do no harm," homeopathy is a safe and effective system of treating many common acute and chronic ailments. Homeopathic remedies are nontoxic; in more than two hundred years of using these formulations, there have been no reported cases of a permanent adverse reaction.

Homeopathic Treatment

For temporary insomnia, you can treat yourself with homeopathic remedies after consulting with your doctor. You can obtain remedies from homeopathic pharmacists, or even from some drugstores or health food stores. For chronic insomnia, you should consult a qualified homeopathic practitioner. Professional homeopathic medical doctors graduate from conventional four-year medical schools with a doctor of nmedicine (M.D.) degree and often complete postgraduate training in homeopathy to learn this holistic specialty. To find a trained homeopathic practitioner, you can contact the National Center for Homeopathy listed in Section 50; they can give you a referral to a practitioner in your area.

Homeopathic doctors agree that chronic sleep problems require constitutional, professional treatment. But the short-term remedies below may help break the sleep-cycle problem and put you on the right track. If no improvement is noticed within three weeks, consult your doctor or homeopath before continuing the treatment.

General instructions for all remedies. Take the recommended remedy one hour before going to bed for ten nights running; repeat dose if woken by a nightmare or if you wake and cannot get to sleep again.

- For sleeplessness due to great mental irritability or overindulgence in food or alcohol, if you wake around three or four A.M., then fall asleep just as it is time to get up: *Nux vomica*
- If you yawn a lot but cannot sleep; if you experience light sleeping, especially after emotional upset; if you have nightmares when you do sleep: *Ignatia*
- If you experience sleeplessness with anxiety and restlessness; if you wake between midnight and two A.M.; if sleeplessness worsens when you are overtired: *Arsenicum album*
- If you experience sleeplessness from aches and pains; if you feel irritable, restless and walk about; if your symptoms worsen after midnight: *Rhus tox*

#29

CONSIDER ACUPUNCTURE

Licensed acupuncturist Annie Reibel of New York City says that insomnia can be caused by an imbalance of body energy. She believes that acupuncture can be very helpful in returning this balance.

Acupuncture is one part of an Oriental medical system developed in China. The ancient Chinese believed that we are born with a finite amount of energy circulation in our bodies, called *chi* or *qu*. The *chi* flows from one meridian into the other, completing an energy cycle every twenty-four hours; it is a dynamic force that gives us life. But stresses such as extreme moods, weather conditions, eating or drinking habits, or too much or too little sex or exercise can disrupt the flow of *chi* in different parts of the body. The purpose of acupuncture is to stimulate points on the body's energy meridians to unblock stuck *chi*, speed it up if it is flowing too slowly, or slow it down if it is racing too fast. By inserting and manipulating needles in the correct energy points, the excess or deficiency in the *chi* that causes insomnia can be rebalanced.

Acupuncturists say that in the daytime there's a relative outward movement of *chi* and blood toward the muscles that returns inward during sleep to nourish the internal organs. Insomnia results when the energy cannot easily return to a restful place or when the internal organs (usually the heart or kidneys) cannot hold on to that energy for the duration of the night. There are certain organs in the body that serve to promote this calming and nurturing function; influencing these organs through acupuncture can help a person fall asleep and stay asleep. For those who can't fall asleep, the acupuncturist may look to calm an agitated liver; those who suffer late-night awakenings may need manipulation of the energy flow through the heart or kidneys.

METHODS OF TREATMENT

Acupuncture needles are inserted quickly and left in place for several minutes. Sometimes the practitioner just pierces the skin, while other times the needle is inserted up to an inch deep. The practitioner may twirl the needle to increase stimulation. Another process of stimulating the acupuncture points is called moxabustion. In one method of moxabustion, the needles' heads are wrapped with dry moxa (Chinese wormwood) and burned. The needle conducts the heat into the acupuncture point. In yet another process, called electroacupuncture, the practitioner connects each needle to a small machine that stimulates the needles with a low electrical pulse.

The chosen method of treatment depends on the acupuncturist's view of what is causing the insomnia, where the flow of *chi* is disrupted, and what will best restore balance.

The Course of Treatment

Reibel has found that most insomniacs find relief after just two or three acupuncture treatments. Naturally, the course of treatment depends on the root cause of the insomnia. You can help the acupuncturist make a correct diagnosis and determine the best plan of therapy if you evaluate your state of sleep hygiene (as explained in Chapter Two) before your visit. What is your daily sleep schedule? Do you smoke? Drink too much coffee or alcohol? Take medications? Feel depressed or stressed? All of these factor into the correct placement of the acupuncture needles. The success of the treatments and their lasting effect depend on the individual's willingness to alter the habits that are affecting the body's energy flow. When combined with positive lifestyle changes, just a few acupuncture sessions can have a lifelong effect on insomnia.

Finding an Acupuncturist

Acupuncture for insomnia is most effective when properly administered with a correct diagnosis; that's why it's important to find a skilled practitioner. Licensing of acupuncturists varies by state: Some license independent practitioners, while others restrict practice to medical doctors (those with an M.D.) or allow acupuncturists to work only under such a doctor's supervision. For information regarding licensing requirements in your state and for help finding a licensed therapist in your area, contact the National Commission for Certification of Acupuncturists listed in Section 50.

Reibel suggests that the effects of acupuncture on insomnia can be enhanced when the treatment is combined with herbal therapy (see Section 27). Because insomnia is generally caused by a physical imbalance, acupuncture is a highly effective treatment in restoring that balance—and restful sleep.

#30

ADMINISTER ACUPRESSURE

Acupressure is a therapy similar to acupuncture in that it uses the same geography of meridians and pressure points. Instead of using needles, however, a practitioner or the individual himself uses hands or feet to gently pressure the appropriate points. Acupressure relaxes tense muscles, improves blood circulation, and stimulates the body's ability to relax deeply and fall asleep.

The advantage of acupressure's healing touch is that it is safe to do on yourself and others, even if you've never done it before. There are no side effects from drugs, and the only equipment you need are your two hands.

ACUPRESSURE POINTS FOR INSOMNIA

Basically, four pressure points are used to relieve insomnia: points on both heels, the point underneath the base of the skull, the one directly between the eyebrows, and one on the inside of the wrist. Those who have applied acupressure to these points have reported that they not only sleep more deeply without waking, they also tend to feel more alert and have greater energy the following day.

The following acupressure points are suggested by Michael Reed Gach, author of *Acupressure's Potent Points*. You do not have to use all of these points. Try them all and use only the ones you feel comfortable doing and which you find effective.

Heel
Joyful Sleep

Location: Directly below the inside of the anklebone in a slight indentation

Benefits: Relieves insomnia, heel and ankle pain, hypertension and anxiety

Calm Sleep

Location: In the first indentation directly below the outer anklebone

Benefits: Relieves insomnia and the back pain that makes it difficult to sleep

Skull
Wind Mansion

Location: In the center of the back of the head in a large hollow under the base of the skull

Benefits: Relieves insomnia as well as mental stress

Forehead
Third Eye Point

Location: Directly between the eyebrows, in the indentation where the bridge of the nose meets the forehead

Benefits: Relaxes the central nervous system for relieving anxiety and insomnia

Wrist
Spirit Gate

Location: On the inside of the wrist crease, in line with the little finger
Benefits: Relieves anxiety, cold sweats, and insomnia originating from overexcitement

APPLYING ACUPRESSURE

To apply acupressure, use prolonged finger pressure directly on the point. Gradual, steady penetrating pressure for approximately three minutes is ideal. Apply and release finger pressure gradually because this allows the tissues time to respond, promoting healing. Then slowly decrease the finger pressure, ending with about twenty seconds of light touch.

For best results, you should perform the acupressure routines daily and continue using the same points even after you've obtained relief to prevent recurrence of your insomnia. If you cannot practice every day, treating yourself to acupressure two or three times a week can still be effective.

When you begin, you may find that you are most comfortable holding a point for two to three minutes. You can gradually work up to holding points longer, but do not hold any one point longer than ten minutes.

CAUTION

- Use only gentle pressure; it should not cause any pain.
- Pregnant women should use acupressure only under the instruction of a qualified acupuncture or acupressure practitioner.

• Do not use acupressure when taking any drugs or alcohol.
• Do not administer immediately after eating.

You can enhance the power of acupressure to restore sleep by pressing a point and visualizing yourself getting sleepy while you breathe deeply. This will help you realize the full potential power of each pressure point.

#31

CONSIDER CHIROPRACTIC CARE

The word *chiropractic* means "treatment by the hands, or manipulation." It is a system of healing that was developed by David Daniel Palmer (1845–1913) in Iowa in 1895. Palmer believed that displacements of the spine caused pressure on nerves, which created pain or symptoms in other parts of the body.

Dr. Brian Fradet, a member of the Foundation for Chiropractic Education and Research, says that as a direct course of treatment, chiropractic is not appropriate therapy for insomnia. But, he says, it may be very helpful in remedying the imbalances that may be causing sleepless nights.

HOW CHIROPRACTIC CARE CAN HELP

It's very often strained and stressed nerves that rob us of sleep. Through manual manipulation of your spinal cord the chiropractor is able to reduce stress on the central nervous system that may be inhibiting your ability to relax fully.

Chronic pain too may contribute to sleepless nights, and in these cases chiropractic treatment is often a highly effective natural remedy. Studies in North America, Europe, and Australia report that approximately 80 percent of chiropractic practice is for musculoskeletal pain, with low-back and neck pain the most common complaints. Another 10 percent is for headache and migraine pain. Chiropractic treatments can also ease the discomfort of neuralgias, general muscular ailments that cause postural defects and fatigue, and functional disorders of the internal organs and systems that are caused by irritation of nerve pathways. If any of these complaints are keeping you awake at night, you might want to consider chiropractic care.

FINDING A CHIROPRACTOR

An experienced doctor should be chosen through a medical or personal recommendation because chiropractic treatment involves highly specific adjustment of the spinal tissues. Always be certain that your chiropractor is state licensed and reputable. Never allow a "paraprofessional" or other unlicensed person attempt to manipulate your spine; this could worsen your problem rather than help. You can get a referral to a trained chiropractor in your area by contacting the American Chiropractic Association listed in Section 50.

No responsible chiropractor will claim to cure your insomnia, but clinical experience and scientific studies suggest that problems originating in the spine play an important role in many physical and mental conditions that rob us of sleep.

#32

TRY THERAPEUTIC TOUCH

Therapeutic touch works on the premise that in a healthy person there's an equilibrium between inward and outward energy flow. We know this energy exists and extends beyond the skin because it is visible through a technique of ultraviolet photography called Kirlian photography. Practitioners of therapeutic touch believe some sleep disorders are caused by an imbalance in this energy field or a disruption in the energy flow. Insomnia can be successfully treated with therapeutic touch as an adjunct to other relaxation techniques.

A NEW THERAPY

Therapeutic touch is a relatively new treatment therapy. It was developed twenty-four years ago by Dora Kunz and Dolores Krieger, R.N., Ph.D. It derives in part from the ancient practice of healing through the laying on of hands, but in therapeutic touch the practitioner doesn't actually touch the recipient. In fact, the recipient doesn't have to believe in therapeutic touch, or be conscious, for that matter, for the outcome to be successful.

The popularity of this treatment has steadily grown since 1975, when Dr. Krieger introduced a graduate nursing course on the practice at New York University. Today therapeutic touch is being taught to hospital nursing staffs around the world and is part of the curriculum at eighty universities in the United States and abroad.

Rochelle B. Mackey, clinical director of the Body/Mind Medical Institute at Morristown Memorial Hospital in New Jersey, believes that insomniacs tend to have negative thought patterns that create negative patterns of energy throughout the body. This stops the body's ability to fall into a restful, natural sleep. The goal of therapeutic touch in the treatment of this sleep disorder is to restore balance to the patient's energy field, which creates a sense of calm and relaxation. Mackey says, "During the treatment my patients often remark on the sense of peace, tranquility, and trust that they feel. Some have been surprised to feel heat permeating them when my hands aren't even touching them."

SCIENTIFIC SUPPORT

A pilot study by Drs. Quinn and Strelkauskas explored various psychologic and immunologic effects of therapeutic touch. The study included four recently bereaved individuals who completed questionnaires designed to measure baseline anxiety, and blood was drawn for baseline immunologic analysis. Anxiety scores for the four subjects was 29 percent lower following treatment with therapeutic touch. (Subjects treated by more experienced practitioners showed a 68 percent increase in the effect of the treatment!) Post-treatment serum analysis also revealed that the percentage of a certain kind of immune suppressor cells had declined in all patients. The results suggest that therapeutic touch may significantly reduce anxiety and bolster the immune system. Both of these effects enhance sleep.

How It Works

Therapeutic touch practitioners facilitate healing by using the hands to consciously direct an energy exchange. Let's take an example. Thirty-five-year-old Helen McMurley lies fully clothed on a table in a small treatment room. The practitioner's hands are positioned apart, one on each side of Helen and about two to six inches from her face. Then, with complete concentration on the patient, the practitioner moves her hands slowly toward Helen's feet, scanning the energy field. There are cues that signify congestion. A healthy, balanced energy field has a smooth, flowing texture and is symmetrical. Signs of imbalance (congestion or deficiency) may include differences from one side of the body to the other in temperature, texture, rhythm, or energy flow. When congestion is found, the practitioner uses a sweeping hand motion known as "unruffling" to free the bound energy.

The treatment takes about fifteen to twenty minutes; when it's finished, Helen feels completely relaxed and ready to sleep. She laughs, "Too bad I can't bring you home with me so I can fall asleep tonight." The practitioner then explains that the next step for Helen is to learn how to re-create that same feeling at home.

Self-help

Before insomniacs like Helen can mentally re-create the calm of therapeutic touch, they need the help of a professional practitioner to feel the energy patterns and recognize when they're blocked. Once this is felt, the patient can be taught to re-create the feeling of balanced energy with cognitive therapies such as meditation and/or visualization.

These are powerful tools for reestablishing energy flow within the field.

For the treatment of insomnia Mackey likes to meet with patients once a week for about ten weeks. By this time the patient has learned to re-create the state of relaxation and balance energy herself and no longer needs the professional help or regularly scheduled therapeutic touch sessions.

Finding a Therapeutic Touch Practitioner

You can find a therapeutic touch practitioner who is professionally trained by contacting Nurse Healers Professional Associates, Inc. (listed in Section 50) and asking for a therapist in your area.

#33

EXPLORE MASSAGE

It is unlikely that massage alone can cure insomnia. But when combined with relaxation exercises, it can be very effective. There is much evidence that a person's state of mind and the condition of the nervous system is reflected in the muscles of the body, so anything that relaxes the muscles works wonders in calming the mind and the nervous system. That's why massage can effectively break the tension cycle of insomnia.

If you decide to give massage a try, be careful: Massage can be either sedating or stimulating to the body. That's why you should tell a massage therapist that you want a massage that will help you overcome insomnia. A trained and skilled practitioner can tailor a session to treat insomnia by reducing muscular tension and promoting relaxation.

It's hard to say exactly which kind of massage is best for insomnia. Most skilled practitioners do not use just one style or one particular stroke, but a combination of a variety of techniques. Licensed therapist Julia Cowan, who is the teaching staff director at the Atlanta School of Massage, says that a Swedish massage, for example, tends to be relaxing for most people, but the effect on each individual depends on the application, the duration of the treatment, the particular amount of time spent on a specific body part, the pressure, and the other strokes combined with it. It takes a trained and sensitive therapist to cue in to your personal needs.

How Often?

During your first session your therapist will interview you to determine the type and frequency of treatment that you both decide is appropriate. Cowan says, "I prefer to see my clients once a week for a period of four weeks, and then together we assess their progress and decide on a plan of action for the future."

Relaxation Techniques

To get the most benefit from massage, a therapist will encourage an awareness of mind-body balance and will probably suggest the use of other tools to help you consciously relax. Along with massage, you can gain additional benefits if you use relaxation techniques like focused breathing or guided imagery (see Section 36). In fact, the effectiveness of massage to treat insomnia relies on the client's willingness to practice relaxation therapies every day. This helps develop the habit of addressing the body-mind tension that's keeping you awake. If you have an agitated mind, the tension in your body is not going to let you drift off. Daily relaxation exercises will enhance the benefit of the time allotted for a massage and contribute to the long-term benefits. Massage and relaxation techniques enhance total well-being; this in turn helps the body to regulate itself in the normal patterns of sleep, rest, and awake time.

CAUTION

Although there are many benefits from therapeutic body massage, there are situations in which particular manipulations may do more harm than good. A medical professional must always be consulted if there is any doubt regarding the advisability of therapy, since contraindications are unique to each client.

The following is a list of conditions, compiled by therapist Cowan, for which almost any type of massage is always contraindicated:

- osteoporosis or brittle bones
- abnormal body temperature
- acute infectious diseases or systemic infections
- acute inflammatory conditions
- severe high blood pressure or history of heart failure
- skin problems (affected area only)

A primary-care provider should be consulted for advice prior to receiving massage therapy if you have any of these conditions:

- varicose veins, phlebitis, thrombosis (superficial massage around these areas may be very helpful)
- pregnancy (massage in low-risk and uncomplicated pregnancies is appropriate if performed by trained pregnancy massage therapist)
- edema (massage is contraindicated if swelling is the result of heart or kidney disease, obstruction of lymph channels, or toxemia)
- specific conditions or diseases (severe asthma, diabetes, cancer, etc.)
- chronic pain or dysfunction of the muscular or skeletal system

- chronic fatigue (massage over a period of time may help to restore energy once the possibility of disease has been ruled out)
- during use of medication and drugs

Find an Experienced and Trained Therapist

It's very important that your massage therapist is skillfully trained—so do not use the yellow pages as your guide to finding a practitioner. Inconsistencies in national accreditation and licensing make it difficult to obtain a guarantee that everyone listed in the phone book is really a trained therapist. Some states, such as Florida, require that professional massage practitioners earn a certificate from a five-hundred-hour approved school. (A massage certificate may also qualify a practitioner's services for medical insurance reimbursement if the client is referred by a primary-care provider.) Unfortunately, some local governments mistakenly classify massage with escort services and require massage therapists to register with the police and have their fingerprints taken when they apply for a massage business license. Other states have no educational or business regulations at all.

There are two safe ways to find a good massage therapist:

1. Call the American Massage Therapy Association (AMTA, listed in Section 50). This association, which promotes massage therapy, has grown from a handful of members in the 1940s to more than 23,000 professionals today with chapters in every state. A representative can put you in touch with therapists who are AMTA members in your area.
2. Use the yellow pages to locate a school of massage whose programs are approved or accredited by the AMTA's Commission of Massage Training Accredi-

tation/Approval. A representative from one of these schools can head you in the right direction. Schools are an important source of information because not all trained and qualified massage practitioners belong to the American Massage Therapy Association.

CHAPTER SIX

CREATE A PERSONALIZED SLEEP PROGRAM

#34

REARRANGE YOUR SLEEP
ENVIRONMENT

There are no steadfast rules governing your sleep environment. Most of us arrange our bedrooms based purely on personal preference. But it could be that your sleep environment is what's affecting the quality of your sleep. Take a few minutes to evaluate your bedroom and determine if there are changes you can make to help you get a good night's sleep.

BED AND BEDDING

If your mattress is lumpy, sagging, or causing you discomfort, get rid of it and think carefully about the kind of mattress you want to replace it. Mattresses are available in three different types: innerspring, foam, and waterbed.

Innerspring mattresses support the body with coils. The firmness of the mattress is dependent on the thickness of the wire coils and the amount of turns in each coil.

A foam mattress supports the body with foam. If you prefer sleeping on foam rather than on coils but still want support, remember the heavier the foam, the higher the density, therefore the better the support. If you want comfort as well as support, buy a foam mattress that offers a dense inner core surrounded by a soft outer layer.

Waterbeds are another story. Some sleepers are nauseated by the motion associated with a waterbed; others find it relaxing. Most experts agree that the "waveless" type of waterbed with built-in baffles, a liner, and a heater is preferable.

If you suspect that your insomnia is the result of back pain, especially low-back pain, you may want to switch to a firmer mattress. Another way to gain support is to place a bed board between your box spring and mattress. Also, sleep researchers have found that a mattress pad of sheep's wool can decrease movements during the night as well as relieve morning stiffness associated with arthritis.

If you wake in the morning with a stiff neck, you should try sleeping on a soft down pillow that assumes the shape of your head and neck. Sleeping on a contoured pillow will achieve the same effect if you prefer sleeping on foam rather than feathers. If you frequently awake during the night with heartburn or if you experience difficulty in breathing, you should sleep with your head elevated above your feet. Simply raise the head of the bed with wooden blocks, or fold a blanket or two under the head of the mattress, or sleep on a wedge-shaped pillow or several pillows.

Use sheets made of cotton rather than synthetic or satin ones. Cotton sheets breathe, absorb moisture, and create less static electricity, which gives you a more comfortable rest.

If you sleep with a bed partner and you are constantly jostling for bed space during the night, you may need to buy a larger bed that can better accommodate you and your partner. Some insomniacs sleep best with two twin mattresses placed atop a king-size frame. When one person rolls over with this arrangement, movement of the mattress doesn't disturb the other.

Noise and Light

Once you have a comfortable bed, you have to decide where you're going to put it. For most sleepers a dark, quiet room is preferred for a good night's sleep. Some people adjust well to changes in their sleep environment, while others (especially elderly sleepers and insomniacs) are disturbed by the slightest change in their surroundings.

Wake-up thresholds vary with each individual. Some people are awakened by a soft noise like a whisper, while others need to be exposed to a much louder noise. In addition, women and the elderly tend to be more sensitive to noise than men and younger people. It is not only sheer volume but the nature of the noise that arouses sleepers. A mother, for example, is more likely to be awakened by her baby's crying than by a thunderstorm.

Sensitivity to sound is also dependent on the stage of sleep the sleeper is in. A sleeper who is in the lighter stages is more likely to be disturbed by noise than one in the deeper stages. As the need for sleep increases, the wake-up threshold increases as well. An individual who has been deprived of sleep is more difficult to arouse because sleep that follows sleep deprivation is very deep.

A frequently cited study conducted in Los Angeles yielded some interesting results concerning noise and how it disturbs sleep. People who lived close to a busy airport were interviewed regarding their sleep quality. The majority said they had grown accustomed to the sounds of planes flying overhead and that their sleep did not suffer. After the interviews researchers evaluated their sleep by monitoring brain waves. Using recording electrodes connected to transmitters, they received the signals in a receiving truck parked in the subjects' driveways. Although the majority of those interviewed reported that they were not disturbed by the noise of incoming and outgoing flights, researchers discovered that they actually awoke frequently when airplanes flew over. Those who lived close to the airport were getting about forty-five to sixty minutes less sleep and less deep sleep than those living farther away.

If your sleep is easily disturbed by noise, you can take some measures to make your sleep environment more sound-proof:

- Use heavy draperies and carpeting to absorb noise.
- Use earplugs.
- Mask sleep-disturbing sounds with white noise. This is any low-frequency, steady, and monotonous sound. You can purchase a white-noise machine or simply run a fan, an air conditioner, or tune your radio to the static between stations.
- Listen to quiet music while you're trying to fall asleep.
- Try tapes and CDs that capture the sound of rain forests, the ocean, whales, or any other sound of nature that you find soothing.

Many sleepers are disturbed by light that pervades their eyelids when they have their eyes closed. If you are one of these people, you should hang room-darkening shades or heavy draperies on your windows to block out unwanted light. If light still bothers you, try a sleeping mask.

BEDROOM CLOCKS

Most experts agree that the bedroom should be a time-free environment. If you're in the habit of staring at your clock while you're trying to fall asleep, or if you check the clock every time you roll over during the night, put it out of sight. Set the alarm and hide the clock in a drawer or put it on the floor next to your bed where it cannot be seen.

TEMPERATURE AND AIR QUALITY

The ideal sleeping temperature is between 64 and 70 degrees Fahrenheit. When the temperature rises above 75 degrees, sleepers tend to become restless; their sleep becomes shallow, and they experience frequent awakenings. In addition, if your home or apartment is artificially heated, you may experience itchy, dry skin, a dry and scratchy throat, or a stuffed nose; all of these will further disturb your sleep.

To improve your chances of sleeping through the night, lower the heat and try running a humidifier during the night. This will ease the effects of these sleep zappers.

Beds, bedding, noise, light, clocks, temperature, and air quality all make up your sleep environment. Experiment with each until you find a comfort level that will ease you into a good night's sleep.

35

Stop Trying to Sleep

If you have the tendency to fall asleep during sedentary activities (like watching television or reading), but the act of climbing into bed makes you feel wide awake, then there is a possibility that the anxiety caused by the fear of not being able to sleep may be causing your insomnia. Many insomniacs have developed what is known as psychophysiological insomnia, in which they have conditioned themselves to view their bed as a battleground. When you become anxious about sleeplessness, you start a vicious cycle. The more anxious you become about whether you're going to sleep or not, the more aroused you become. The more aroused you become, the less likely it is you will sleep. The less sleep you get, the more anxious you become about what effect this will have on you and your ability to get to sleep the next night, and you're off and running in circles.

Like digestion, heart rate, respiration, or perspiration, sleep is an involuntary function of the autonomic nervous system. When you try to activate these systems yourself, the body becomes aroused, which pushes sedation and ultimately sleep further away. As you lie in bed thinking, "I have to sleep. I need to sleep," or, "How am I going to feel tomorrow if I don't sleep?" you put pressure on yourself. The more you try to control something that cannot be controlled, the more your body is aroused, causing anxiety. Anxiety that started in your mind may now be evident in physiological signs like increased heart rate, shortness of breath, restlessness, and perspiration.

People who are likely to develop psychophysiological insomnia are those who are accustomed to being in control of events in their lives. They are individuals who tend to be sought by others during times of crisis or emergency. Experts believe that one night of sleeplessness may cause these kinds of individuals to feel that they are losing control. This loss of control may lead to ego deflation and possibly psychophysiological insomnia.

WHAT CAN I DO TO STOP MYSELF FROM TRYING TO SLEEP?

To call a truce in your sleeptime battle, you might try a stimulus-control therapy known as the Bootzin Technique, developed by Dr. Richard Bootzin while he was at Northwestern University in Chicago. The Bootzin Technique requires that you use your bed for only two activities: sleep and sex. You go to bed only when you are sleepy, and then if you are unable to fall asleep after trying for fifteen minutes, you get out of bed and move into another room. (If you live in a studio apartment, get out of bed and sit in a chair.) Once in the other room, perform a sedentary activity such as reading, watching television, or working on a calming hobby or craft. No smoking, eating, or exercising. Lights should be as low as possible, and if it is dawn or if you are a night-shift worker sleeping days, draw the shades or blinds to prevent excess light from entering the room. To discourage yourself from getting back into bed too soon, do not time your activities. Go back to bed only when you can no longer keep your eyes open. Dr. Donn Posner at Brown Medical School tells his patients: "Don't get out of bed with the idea that you'll ultimately return to bed that night. The job of someone who is trying to overcome the idea of fighting to fall asleep is to give up. When you get out of bed, I want you to think that you're not going to sleep the rest of the night. Any sleep you get the rest of the night is gravy. You're done. If you get no sleep, so be it; tomorrow's another day. Maybe you'll get some sleep tomorrow." Over time, with consistency, this mind-set may eliminate the struggle and anxiety you've associated with trying to fall asleep.

You might also try a type of sleep restriction that Dr. Arthur Spielman of City College in New York uses to help his patients sleep more soundly. He asks his patients to decrease the time they spend in bed. For example, if you go to bed at ten and wake at six, but spend only about four of those eight hours asleep, you really should be spending only four hours in bed. Spielman suggests that people with this particular schedule might go to bed at 2:00 A.M. and rise at 6:00 A.M. As his patients' sleep efficiency rates (hours spent asleep divided by the hours spent in bed) increase, he allows them to go to bed earlier and earlier each night. This program enables patients to regain the confidence that they have lost in their ability to sleep. Under these types of conditions, people tend to sleep more soundly because no matter how anxious they are, when they get into bed they're really tired and ready to sleep.

Many experts agree that the bedroom should be a time-free environment. If you are in the habit of watching the seconds tick away while trying to fall asleep or if you look at the clock instantly upon waking in the middle of the night to see exactly how long you've slept, it's time to hide your bedroom clock. You should set your alarm as usual, but then hide your clock where it cannot be seen. A clock in the bedroom often raises an insomniac's anxiety level.

If you are not sleeping because you have conditioned yourself to view your bed as a battleground, it's time to surrender. Only when you stop trying to sleep will you begin to get some sleep.

#36

LEARN RELAXATION TECHNIQUES

As you've learned, stress and anxiety can cause sleeplessness. In this section we will look at some relaxation techniques that can help relieve your body of the tension which interferes with a good night's sleep. You don't have to do all the techniques to benefit. Give each one a try and choose the ones you're most comfortable with.

HOW DO I CHOOSE A RELAXATION TECHNIQUE?

Choose a technique that targets the area of your body in which you feel the most tension. For example, if you have shortness of breath, a tightness in the chest, and a racing heart, then abdominal breathing might prove most beneficial. If your neck, shoulders, and back are tense, then muscle relaxation might do the trick. If your mind races from thought to thought, affecting your ability to concentrate, then a meditation or mental-imagery technique may be best for you.

The most effective way to locate stress is to scan your

body for tension. Before you begin, make yourself as comfortable as possible. Remove your shoes, loosen any tight-fitting clothing, loosen your belt, and take off any jewelry that may distract you. Now you are ready to locate hidden tension.

Lie down or sit comfortably in a chair that supports your head. Close your eyes if it helps you focus your attention. In your mind begin to scan your body, searching for tension or tightness. Start with your head and scan all the way down to your feet. Look for tightness in your neck, shoulders, and jaw. See if your teeth are clenched or if your spine is rigid. Notice your pulse. Check your breathing. Is it shallow rather than deep? Scan your stomach for nervousness, cramping, or nausea. Check to see if your toes are curled.

Once the trouble spots have been located, you can choose one or several of the following techniques to calm your body and prepare it for sound sleep.

Relaxation Techniques

Abdominal Breathing

Voluntary control of breathing has been used for centuries to reduce stress and anxiety. To begin, lie down or sit comfortably in a chair that supports your head. Breathe normally, observing the rhythm. Then begin deep breathing:

- Put your hand on your stomach.
- Take a deep breath from the bottom of your stomach.
- Feel it fill you with warm air.
- Feel your hand rise with your stomach muscles.
- Breathe in as you silently count to five.
- Let the air go. Don't push it out. Let it go gently to the count of five.
- When you let out the air, smile.

- Do this sequence two times in a row.
- Then breathe regularly (rhythmically and comfortably).
- Breathe deeply again after you have let a minute or two go by.
- Repeat this deep-breathing/regular-breathing cycle two or three times, or as often as needed.

Progressive Muscle Relaxation

When a muscle is tensed for a few seconds and then released, it is easier to identify the tension in that muscle and compare it to its relaxed state. "It's also a classical conditioning paradigm," says Dr. Posner. "You are repeatedly pairing tension followed by relaxation, which you hope ultimately occurs naturally over time. As you become tense, your body's next response is relaxation."

Lie down or sit in a comfortable chair that supports your head. Focus your attention on your right hand. Clench it into a fist, squeezing it as hard as you can for about five seconds. Open the fist and allow your muscles to relax. Observe the difference between your right hand, which is now in a deeply relaxed state, and your left hand, which is in its natural state. You should notice a profound difference. Repeat the exercise, then do the same for the left hand. Repeat the exercise for the muscles in your arms, face, neck, shoulders, abdomen, buttocks, thighs, calves, and feet.

Passive Relaxation

Once you have mastered the tense-and-release technique of relaxation, you can move on to passive relaxation. In this method you focus on the individual muscle groups as you did in the tense-and-release method; however, you omit the tensing phase of the exercise. Rather, direct your attention to the muscle group and recall the feeling of deep relaxation that came over your muscles naturally after tensing. In your mind's eye, see the muscles relaxing, feel the release of tension. Watch the blood flow freely and smoothly through the muscles. Concentrate on their fluid and relaxed state. Imagining it can make it happen.

Meditation and Yoga

In the last moments before sleep onset the brain emits alpha waves. The state of passive concentration produced by meditation has the same effect on the brain. Meditation helps to decrease the activity of the sympathetic nervous system, reducing tension and anxiety, slowing respiration and heart rate, and lowering blood pressure.

During meditation your mind and body are quieted through concentration. For example, if you practice Zen meditation you concentrate on breathing; if you practice Transcendental meditation you concentrate on a mantra (a calming word or phrase). Other types of meditation require you to focus on an object such as a flame of a candle, a leaf, or still water. In prayerful meditation you concentrate on communication on a spiritual level.

Yoga is a form of relaxation that originated in India. It consists of physical and mental disciplines that tend to the needs of the whole body. Through breathing, positions, and postures called *asanas*, yoga can also address specific body parts.

Meditation and yoga are relaxation techniques that should be learned from a trainer. Many colleges, adult education centers, and dance studios offer classes in meditation and yoga. Consult your yellow pages for the ones nearest you.

Mental Imagery

It is said that the mind never thinks without a picture. Sights, smell, sounds, and touch are all included in mental images. The images that pervade your mind affect the way you feel as well as the way your body behaves physiologically. Images serve as cues stimulating the nervous system, causing muscles to respond subconsciously. Mental imagery, probably one of the oldest relaxation techniques known, can allow you to achieve a relaxation response.

Lie down or sit comfortably in a chair that supports your head. Close your eyes and allow your mind to create a relaxing scene. The scene you create should be one you are familiar with, one you find relaxing. Put yourself in the scene. Be sure to hear the sounds, smell the smells, experience the sensations. For example, you may want to create a scene in which you are walking through the woods. Feel the moisture in the air from the lush, green vegetation. Notice the grass beneath your bare feet. Smell the blooming flowers. See the insects gathering pollen. Hear the birds and cicadas, listen for the gentle breeze rustling the leaves.

If you do not find the woods a relaxing place, then imagine yourself bathed in afternoon sunlight on a tropical beach or in the park down the street. Imagine yourself in any scene that is comforting and relaxing and which you can retreat to quickly and easily when you feel stress.

Biofeedback

Biofeedback teaches you to control physiological functions such as heart rate, muscle tension, blood pressure, blood flow, and brain waves under the supervision of trained health-care professionals. While your body is being monitored by biofeedback instruments, you hear a gentle tone. As your body begins to tense, the tone's pitch increases. You learn how to use relaxation techniques to relax your body and lower the pitch of the tone. This enables you to learn which mental states bring on tension and which ones calm it.

WHEN SHOULD I DO RELAXATION TECHNIQUES?

It is very important to practice relaxation techniques and learn them well before attempting to use them at bedtime to ward off sleeplessness. A failed attempt to relax at bedtime causes more anxiety and can condition you to associate relaxation techniques with insomnia. Set aside a time of day to work on your relaxation exercises. It is imperative that you make a distinction between practice and use. "I like to tell my patients that muscle relaxation, breathing, or any of those things should be considered skills not unlike driving a car, or swinging a baseball bat, or learning to play a musical instrument," says Dr. Posner. "When we think about any of these skills, what we tend to do with them is practice them when we don't need them. We practice piano at home, not in front of a concert audience; we practice driving a car on a quiet street, not on a highway." Practice relaxation techniques while you are completely calm. Then you can focus on the effects of relaxation rather than the technique itself.

#37

Exercise!

Exercise is one of the key components of sleep hygiene (the lifestyle and dietary habits that promote good sleep). When combined with other components, exercise can help reduce the incidence of insomnia. During vigorous exercise the brain generates chemicals called endorphins. These chemicals are the body's natural painkillers and produce a sense of calm and well-being. Many people do not exercise at all yet sleep fine. On the other hand, those who have a sleep problem and do not exercise may want to add some form of exercise to their daily routine.

How Does Exercise Improve Sleep?

To understand how exercise affects sleep, you must understand the circadian rhythm of the human body. The body's circadian rhythm, or inner clock, is a natural biological pattern that causes core body temperature to rise to a peak and decline to a valley every twenty-four hours. For example, the body temperature of individuals who are awake during the day and sleep during the night peaks in the early evening and bottoms out in the early morning just before waking. People who experience insomnia tend to have a flatter temperature rhythm (a lower peak and a higher valley). Because insomniacs are less alert and less active during the day, their body temperature increases less during the day and decreases less during the night, causing their sleep to become shallow.

Vigorous exercise increases the core body temperature by about two degrees Fahrenheit. Exercise performed in the late afternoon or the early evening will force the body temperature to dip much lower during sleep. A lower temperature brings deeper sleep with fewer awakenings. If exercise is performed too close to bedtime, however, an elevated body temperature may make it difficult to fall asleep, since body temperature must be declining to promote sleep. Some sleep experts say that twenty to thirty minutes of intense exercise six hours before you want to sleep will help.

WHAT TYPE OF EXERCISES SHOULD I DO AND HOW OFTEN?

There are a wide range of exercises to choose from. The key to sticking with an exercise program is picking one that you enjoy. Before you begin any workout, remember to warm up with gentle, moderate exercises first. This raises your body temperature, increases blood flow to make more oxygen available for energy production, and makes your muscles pliant. Be sure to ease into your chosen exercise slowly, avoiding forceful movements that can damage muscles and tendons.

After you have warmed up, begin your exercise. You should perform your chosen exercise continuously for twenty to thirty minutes, raising your heart rate to the aerobic target zone for your age. (An aerobic exercise is one that is designed to stimulate and strengthen the heart and increase lung capacity. It is the form of exercise associated with promoting sound sleep.) Your maximum heart rate is approximately 220 minus your age. Compute 60 percent and 75 percent of this number. Between these two numbers is your aerobic heart rate target zone.

While exercising, pause to determine your heart rate. You do this by taking your pulse for ten seconds, counting the number of beats. Multiply the number of beats by six to get the number of heart beats per minute. If you find that your heart rate is slower than your target range, you need to step up the pace of the exercise and work more vigorously. If your rate is above the target zone, slow down; you may be doing yourself more harm than good.

After you have completed your twenty to thirty minutes of exercise, cool the body down to its resting state by exercising gently and slowly for a few minutes.

Before you begin an exercise program you should seek the advice of a physician. This is especially important for anyone who has been sedentary or who has not engaged in regular vigorous physical activity.

If you feel as though you are too tired to exercise, then exercise is exactly what you need. Performing exercise when you are tired can acutely raise your energy level by improving the flow of oxygen through the body. So, if you are having sleep problems, start exercising!

#38

Reset Your Inner Clock

After her high school reunion, Claudia Krass stayed up reminiscing with a few old friends. Finally at 5:00 A.M. she bid her friends good-bye and headed home. At six (the time Claudia usually awoke) she found herself lying in bed staring at the ceiling, unable to fall asleep. The reason? Claudia's biological clock, which was unaware that she had been awake since six the previous morning, was telling her body it was time to be awake.

What Is Your Inner Clock?

Your inner clock, or biological clock, is responsible for setting your body's circadian (daily) rhythm. Neurons set the clock by causing the body's temperature to increase and decrease over a twenty-four-hour period. This fluctuation in body temperature is directly related to your body's physical performance and your mental alertness. For example, if you are diurnal (meaning you sleep during the night and are awake during the day), your body temperature will reach its peak in the late afternoon or early evening. At this point the mind is at its peak alertness. Your body's low temperature will occur sometime in the middle of the night, at which time your mind's attentiveness is considerably diminished. When your body temperature reaches its highest point, your inner clock reads 12:00 biological time. Even when you stay awake all night, your clock ticks away as usual, causing your body temperature to fall as if you were asleep. What you sometimes perceive as a second wind is only your inner clock increasing your body's temperature, thus increasing your body's performance and mental alertness.

This inner clock can cause sleep problems if it's set on a schedule that doesn't coincide with your sleep-wake schedule. For example, if a person needs eight hours of sleep and has to get up at eight, she'd need to be asleep by midnight. But if she didn't fall asleep until two, it may be because her time of peak alertness is two hours too late for her schedule. Thus, she'd need to reset her inner clock so that she'd start getting sleepy at midnight.

How to Access Your Inner Clock

Dr. Nathaniel Kleitman, a pioneer in the field of sleep research, noted that when the body is forced into a new schedule (from a change in work shift, for example), the body's inner clock will reset itself, causing the body's temperature to drop when the person sleeps and to rise when the person is awake. He concluded that the body's circadian rhythm is adjustable. But how is the clock set?

The circadian rhythm you feel as wakefulness and sleepiness is the result of internal body changes. It works something like the clock on your wall. If you remove the back of the clock, you will see springs and gears and other mechanisms that operate the clock. The movement of the hands on the face of the clock is merely a result of the functioning of the inner mechanisms. Unfortunately, you cannot gain access to your inner clock as easily as the clock on your kitchen wall. You can, however, tell your biological time by reading body temperature and circadian rhythm, which are results of the functioning of your clock's internal mechanisms.

Dr. Michael Bonnet of the Wright State School of Medicine and the director of the Sleep Disorders Center at the Dayton VA Hospital in Dayton, Ohio, treats insomniacs with chronotherapy. To gain access to his patients' individual inner clocks, he asks them to keep a sleep journal (hours slept, wake time, and amount of time taken to fall asleep; see section 6) and to take their temperatures every hour throughout the day. Although accurate temperature readings are needed for only two days, patients must log into their sleep journals every day for three weeks. Sleep journals are a valuable tool in determining if the patient is a long sleeper or a short one. Plotting a patient's temperature provides information on the peaks and valleys of body temperature. By gathering this information Dr. Bonnet can determine if the patient's clock is shifted ahead in time or back in time (if you go to sleep one hour later than usual, you are then living on a twenty-five-hour schedule; one hour earlier, you're on a twenty-three-hour schedule).

RESETTING YOUR INNER CLOCK

Nature provides all living organisms with behavioral and physical cues that help them set their inner clocks. Dr. Bonnet advises his patients who have difficulty falling asleep to use these cues to shift their circadian rhythm to suit their daily schedule. For some this means moving their body's rhythm backward; others move forward. For example, if you want to sleep from twelve to eight but have gotten into a sleep schedule of two to ten, you must move your rhythm back two hours. Your first step in moving your inner clock back is to choose the time you want to wake and set your alarm clock for that time. Waking at this time may be difficult at first, but it will be well worth the effort in the long run. Once you have dragged yourself from your bed, go into the bright sunshine as soon as possible. Bright light is one of the cues provided by nature to help set your clock. Once in the sunshine you should do some form of exercise—walking or jogging are best. Exercise will raise your body temperature, allowing you to adjust to your new circadian rhythm. Finally, in the evening, starting three to four hours before bedtime, it is important that you avoid conflicting cues that affect your rhythm. Lights should be softened and physical activity minimized. Your body must be given a chance to relax and to cool its temperature. "Following this type of regimen for a few days or even a week should be sufficient to move the body rhythm back a couple of hours to make it easier to fall asleep earlier," says Dr. Bonnet.

#39

TRY BRIGHT-LIGHT THERAPY

If you have trouble falling asleep at night because your inner clock is off schedule, early morning sunlight can help reset your circadian rhythm so that by the end of the day, you're tired and ready for sleep. But the problem with morning light therapy is that the sun is not always cooperative. What if you live in Alaska during the winter or in the Pacific Northwest, where it is foggy and overcast so much of the time? Or, what if you have to rise before the sun? How do you get the light that your body needs to adjust its clock? Bright-light therapy may be the answer.

WHAT IS BRIGHT-LIGHT THERAPY?

Bright-light therapy is used as a surrogate for sunshine. It allows an insomniac who cannot get exposure to sunlight to still benefit from the regulating effects of ultraviolet rays. As light enters the retina, it suppresses the release of melatonin (a hormone released by the pineal gland that has been linked to drowsiness). Bright-light therapy was first investigated in 1980, when scientists at the National Institute for Mental Health (NIMH) were approached by a chemist who found himself severely depressed during winter months. He believed his depression was a symptom of the decrease in sunlight that accompanies winter. The scientists at the NIMH, who were working on the relationship between bright light and melatonin, began to treat the chemist with light therapy. As a result of the treatments, the chemist's depression lifted and a new form of depression was discovered: seasonal affect disorder, or SAD. (See Section 44 for more details on SAD.) It was not long after the discovery of bright light's effect on SAD that bright-light therapy was employed to readjust the inner clocks of insomniacs suffering from Advance Sleep Phase Syndrome (early morning awakenings) and Delayed Sleep Phase Syndrome (difficulty falling asleep).

Light Boxes

Insomniacs receiving bright-light therapy are exposed to light provided by a light box. An average light box is roughly twenty-four inches by thirteen inches and weighs less than ten pounds. Although individual light boxes vary, generally a box delivers 10,000 lux* at a distance of two feet from a cool-white fluorescent bulb.

Dr. Michael Stevenson, clinical director of North Valley Sleep Disorders Center in Mission Hills, California, uses bright-light therapy to treat his patients. He does not try to move a patient's rhythm back or forward all at one time. Unless the individual has morning obligations that require a more abrupt change in sleep phase, he prefers to move the

---

* Lux is a unit used to measure illumination and the amount of light that the retina of the eye receives. The lights of a well-lit office generate about 500 to 1,000 lux.

cycle back gradually by advancing the individual's wake-up time every other day by fifteen minutes and exposing the patient to 4,000 lux at a distance of two feet for one to two hours. Patients receiving bright-light therapy need not look directly into the light. They can read, watch television, or snack while they are exposed to the light. Many sleep-disorder clinics rent or lease light boxes to patients, allowing them to become accustomed to bright-light therapy at home before investing in a box of their own.

CANDIDATES FOR BRIGHT-LIGHT THERAPY

This therapy is not for all types of insomniacs. It is a tool that merely assists you in resetting your inner clock, so it will not help if you have a conditioned insomnia. It is really only for those who suffer from Delayed Sleep Phase Syndrome or Advance Sleep Phase Syndrome (see Section 4). If your insomnia is similar to the following examples, you might want to give bright-light therapy a try.

Let's say you typically go to bed Monday through Friday nights at midnight. You toss and turn until two, when you finally fall asleep. When the weekend comes, however, you go to bed at two and fall asleep ten minutes after your head hits the pillow. This means you suffer from Delayed Sleep Phase, and you are a logical candidate for bright-light therapy.

You are also a candidate if you consistently fall asleep shortly after you go to bed, but then awake in the middle of the night, unable to fall back to sleep (Advance Sleep Phase). The treatment of Advance Sleep Phase Syndrome and Delayed Sleep Phase Syndrome differs only in the time of day that the bright-light therapy is scheduled. Treatment for Delayed Sleep Phase is given in the morning shortly after rising for the day. Advance Sleep Phase treatment is given in the afternoon.

Dr. Stevenson says the success of bright-light therapy

depends on the insomniac's motivation, sleep hygiene, and the distance that the insomniac's clock needs to be moved. If you routinely stay up late and then sleep in on the weekends, you are encouraging your clock to move ahead. "Many people can adjust to the transient problem, while others with a longer circadian rhythm have a more difficult time getting back to their normal rhythm. Those people have to make a lifestyle change. They must give up certain habits, or they can lapse to where they were before," says Dr. Stevenson.

GIVE IT A TRY

If you'd like to give bright-light therapy a try, Dr. Quentin Regestein, director of the sleep clinic at Brigham and Women's Hospital in Boston, Massachusetts, suggests you try making your own light box. Simply get two 100 watt light bulbs and put them in a gooseneck lamp. While sitting at a table or desk, position the lamp eight inches from your eyes in the margin of the visual field. Point the lamp downward to illuminate a magazine, book, newspaper, or whatever you would like to read; then begin reading. Dr. Regestein believes the light reflected off the pages is sufficient to have an effect on your inner clock.

CHAPTER SEVEN

CONSIDER OTHER SLEEP DISORDERS

#40

Suspect Sleep Apnea

A person suffering sleep apnea has much in common with an insomniac. Because neither get a good night's sleep their days are filled with drowsiness. But insomnia and sleep apnea are two very different conditions.

What Is Sleep Apnea?

It is estimated that 10 to 30 percent of adults snore and have no serious medical consequences as a result. But snoring loudly and habitually can be an indication of a potentially life-threatening breathing disturbance known as obstructive sleep apnea syndrome. A 1993 prevalence study performed by Dr. Terry Young showed that 4 percent of the male population and 2 percent of the female population had significant night-time breathing disturbances known as apnea, causing daytime sleepiness. What's more, this problem causes more than drowsiness. Dr. J. Nahmias, of the Sleep Disorders Center at Newark Beth Israel Hospital in Newark, New Jersey says,

"Sleep apnea, when it is moderate to severe, is an independent risk factor for high blood pressure, stroke, heart attacks, right and left ventricular heart dysfunction and heart failure, and sudden death in some studies."

The word *apnea* literally translates to "interrupted breathing." Obstructive sleep apnea syndrome is a condition in which frequent and abnormal cessations of breathing occur during sleep. The cessations are followed by brief awakenings as the sleeper gasps for air. Those with apnea are usually unaware that their rest has been disturbed, but it has. Average apneic episodes last twenty-one or twenty-two seconds, and they can occur as many as four hundred to five hundred times a night. (Dr. Nahmias has witnessed a patient cease breathing 181 times in a one-hour period!) Consequently, one who suffers from sleep apnea can spend more time awake than asleep. But unaware that their sleep had been disturbed the previous night, people with apnea cannot figure out why they're so lethargic during the day.

What Are the Symptoms of Sleep Apnea?

The first symptom is loud snoring. If your snoring is so loud that it wakes your bed partner, can be heard in other rooms of the house, and is interrupted by pauses and then gasps for air, there is a good chance that you suffer from sleep apnea. Frequent daytime drowsiness that disrupts work and your personal life is another indication. Forgetfulness, irritability, anxiousness, depression, or difficulty in concentrating may also accompany sleep apnea. It also manifests itself by causing you to wake in the middle of the night, gasping for air and thrashing around in your bed. Morning headaches and a loss of interest in sex have also been linked to the condition.

What Is the Treatment for Apnea?

Several general guidelines should be followed to alleviate sleep apnea. Losing weight and avoiding alcohol can help the problem. Sleeping pills, which tend to depress breathing and worsen the effects of apnea, should also be avoided. Medications that relieve congestion of the nose and throat, however, may help. Also, a change in sleeping position can aid in alleviating apnea. If you follow these basic guidelines and your apnea persists, you may be a candidate for more specific treatments.

Continuous positive airway pressure (CPAP, pronounced *see-pap*) is the most effective therapy for sufferers of sleep apnea. Dr. Michael Thorpy, director of the Sleep-Wake Disorders Center at Montefiore Hospital, Bronx, New York, has found CPAP to be an effective treatment for about 85 percent of his patients. During CPAP therapy an apnea patient wears a mask over the nose during sleep. An air compressor forces air into the airway. The air exerts pressure on the airway, holding it open and allowing the sleeper to breathe normally. Although the success rate is high, about 22 percent of apnea sufferers find the mask too cumbersome and discontinue the therapy. Those who choose to abandon CPAP therapy may look into the various oral appliances that are designed to bring the jaw, tongue, and soft palate forward, thus opening the airway. If your sleep apnea is not relieved by these devices, surgery may be suggested as a last resort.

For more information call the American Sleep Apnea Association, listed in Section 50.

#41

MAKE A NOTE
OF NARCOLEPSY

Jim Murphy, a fifty-year-old financial account executive, falls asleep at his desk and at occasional social affairs. His family thinks he needs to get more sleep at night. Friends worry he's either depressed or getting lazy. Jim himself has no idea why he can't stay awake. The fact is, his problem isn't lack of sleep; it's too much sleep—a condition called narcolepsy.

WHAT IS NARCOLEPSY?

Narcolepsy is a neurological condition that forces a person into sudden uncontrollable attacks of sleep. An estimated 80,000 to 250,000 Americans suffer from this chronic condition, which can be dangerous. Although narcolepsy itself is not life-threatening, because seizures occur without warning, an attack during activities such as driving, swimming, or cooking could be fatal.

WHAT ARE THE SYMPTOMS OF NARCOLEPSY?

There are six symptoms. The first is excessive daytime sleepiness (EDS). Victims of narcolepsy feel tired at times when they should not. They tend to fall asleep during activities that would encourage most people to stay awake—like swimming, riding a bike, or driving. In most cases EDS is the only symptom.

The second symptom of narcolepsy is cataplexy. Cataplexy, which usually develops several years after the onset of daytime sleepiness, is a sudden yet brief attack of muscle weakness. During a cataplexy attack a person loses muscle control in the arms, legs, and face, and may fall to the ground. The eyes remain open, and although the person is conscious and aware, he is unable to speak. Cataplexy is triggered by stress and strong emotion such as laughter, anger, or surprise.

A third symptom is hypnagogic hallucinations. These hallucinations, which occur at the onset of sleep, are auditory and/or visual sensations that are not easily distinguishable from reality. A narcoleptic faced with a hypnagogic hallucination may fantasize that the bedroom is being occupied by demons, murderers, or strange animals.

Sleep paralysis is the fourth symptom. As with cataplexy, sleep paralysis causes the narcoleptic to lose control of muscle tone. Unlike cataplexy, however, sleep paralysis ceases when the narcoleptic is touched. This symptom usually occurs at the onset of sleep or upon waking.

Another symptom that is found in fifty percent of cases is called automatic behavior. During automatic behavior, narcoleptics fall asleep yet continue the activity they were doing before the onset of sleep. These "blackouts" may last for a few seconds, or they may last for several hours. During the episode the person may appear wide awake and reasonably conscious but display rather erratic behavior. Narcoleptics have been known to drive automobiles during these attacks; others remove all the dishes from the cabinets, and some have completely emptied their bookcases. Many do not remember their actions.

Disturbed nighttime sleep is the sixth symptom. Although narcoleptics frequently have a difficult time staying awake during the day, ironically, they have trouble staying asleep throughout the night.

In addition to these six symptoms, narcoleptics can also exhibit lethargy, low motivation, inability to concentrate, and memory loss.

WHAT CAUSES NARCOLEPSY?

The exact cause is unknown. It is thought to be a disorder of the part of the central nervous system that controls sleep and wakefulness. Unlike a person without the disorder, a narcoleptic's nighttime sleep begins with a REM period. Cataplexy, sleep paralysis, and hypnagogic hallucinations are all similar to the loss of muscle control that takes place during a normal sleeper's REM sleep. Lack of muscle tone and dream experiences that accompany REM sleep occur at inappropriate times for someone suffering from narcolepsy. Narcolepsy is not a psychiatric or physiological problem, but rather it is believed to be a genetic one. Research has indicated that narcoleptics have a set of genes that are triggered by unknown factors to cause narcolepsy.

If you exhibit any of the symptoms discussed and suspect that you may have narcolepsy, a visit to a sleep specialist for accurate diagnosis is recommended.

HOW IS NARCOLEPSY TREATED?

Unfortunately, a cure has not yet been discovered. A narcoleptic can, however, lead a relatively normal life by controlling the symptoms of the disorder. If you have been diagnosed with narcolepsy, a sleep specialist will assist you in choosing a treatment plan that will best suit your lifestyle. A combination of medication, lifestyle adjustments, and environmental management will allow you to control your condition.

The American Sleep Disorders Association suggests making the following adjustments:

- Follow a strict sleep-wake schedule. Go to bed and wake up at approximately the same time every day.
- Take short naps once or twice a day as needed.
- Increase your physical activity and avoid boring or repetitive tasks.
- Carefully follow the doctor's instructions regarding medication. Immediately inform the doctor of any changes or problems with medications.

When untreated, narcolepsy can be a dangerous condition. But with proper attention and treatment, people with narcolepsy enjoy a relatively normal life. For more information about narcolepsy, contact the American Narcolepsy Association, listed in Section 50.

#42

WATCH FOR PERIODIC
LIMB MOVEMENT DISORDER

Ben Holtz, a sixty-seven-year-old retiree from Glen Rock, New Jersey, sat at the breakfast table complaining to his wife, Hazel, about his lack of energy.

"I got eight hours' sleep last night," he said, "so why am I so tired?"

"Maybe it was that marathon you ran all night," Hazel said.

"Marathon? What marathon?" Ben asked.

"Your legs never stopped moving; they kicked and jerked all night long. I'm the one who should be complaining."

Ben doesn't know it, but he has a condition called periodic limb movement disorder (PLMD) that disturbs his sleep at night and makes him feel tired during the day. It's a condition often confused with insomnia.

Periodic Limb Movement Disorder

Periodic limb movement disorder (formerly known as nocturnal myoclonus) involves involuntary, disruptive movements of the legs, and sometimes arms, during sleep. The movements occur at regular intervals and involve a rhythmic extension of the big toe coupled with an upward bending of the ankle, knee, or hip. The movements usually appear in the first half of the night during non-REM sleep. (All limb movements are uncommon in REM sleep because the muscles are normally paralyzed to prevent a person from acting out a dream.) PLMD should not be confused with hypnotic jerks, which usually occur when the body moves from wakefulness to sleep and which are sometimes accompanied by the mental image of missing a step. Nocturnal cramps, which can be a delayed reaction to strenuous daytime activities, are also quite different from PLMD.

The complaints of people with PLMD vary, depending on the time of the limb disturbances and how the disturbances are perceived. For example, people who complain of difficulty in falling asleep usually do fall asleep, but they awaken so quickly after sleep onset that they think they've been awake the whole time. People with PLMD may complain that they wake frequently during the night. The awakenings are caused by the "microarousals" that accompany the leg movements. Because some people who have PLMD are not aware that its disruptive limb movements are keeping them awake at night, they will often complain of insomnia. Dr. J. Nahmias says he has many patients who kick so violently during sleep that they are up half the night. Others have no recollection of the sleep disturbances. "If people say they wake up exhausted or that they are falling asleep during the day, you know that the arousals are disturbing sleep," says Dr. Nahmias. This can result in insomnia-like daytime problems.

PLMD rarely occurs in people under 30. And only 5 percent of people ages 30 to 50 are affected by PLMD. From ages 50 to 65, PLMD affects 29 percent of the population; over age 65, 44 percent are likely to be affected by the condition.

DIAGNOSES AND TREATMENTS FOR PLMD

The cause of PLMD is unclear, but the American Sleep Disorders Association reports that 20 percent of those who are diagnosed with insomnia also have PLMD. If you answer yes to any of the following questions, you may have PLMD:

- Does your bed partner complain of being kicked in the night?
- Do you find your bed covers twisted or on the floor in the morning?
- Do you feel sleepy during the day when you think you've had a full night's sleep?
- Do you wake frequently in the night?
- Do you have difficulty falling asleep?

You can see why PLMD is confused with insomnia. If these symptoms sound familiar, or if you have any other reason to suspect that you have PLMD, your sleep should be observed by a sleep-disorders professional.

#43

READ ABOUT RESTLESS LEG SYNDROME

Shirley Bowen has had restless leg syndrome since she was a child. Now in her forties, she recalls that when she went to the movies as a teenager, her date would be sitting watching the film and she would be pacing around the lobby. A few years ago, just before Christmas, Bowen said she went through an entire week during which she had a total of eight hours of sleep and "I really was thinking about suicide."

Like many of the estimated 12 million Americans who suffer from restless leg syndrome (RLS), Shirley's condition was misdiagnosed for years. It's a disorder that's hard to describe. People who experience RLS often describe a "creepy crawly" sensation deep within their legs during relaxation and especially at bedtime. These sensations are usually limited to the lower legs, between the knees and ankles, but can also be experienced in the arms. People with RLS often describe the sensations as being deep in the bones. RLS can be very painful to some. The pain, however, is not like that experienced during leg cramps or when the supply of blood to a limb has been interrupted, causing it to "fall asleep."

For those who experience RLS, relief from the sensations comes only after the legs are moved, which is why the condition is called restless leg syndrome. People with RLS have an irresistible urge to move their legs. When these people get up and move the legs, or stretch them, or massage them, the sensation goes away. As soon as they sit down and relax again, this irresistible urge returns. Unfortunately, this condition causes a loss of sleep that can result in daytime drowsiness.

Research has shown that the syndrome is often familial and is linked to the body's circadian sleep-wake cycles—worsening in the afternoon and evening and disappearing after about three A.M. It gets worse when the individual is sitting down or lying in bed. It can affect children as well as adults, but seems to worsen with age. Men and women are equally affected, but it is rarely seen in the African-American community, according to Richard P. Allen of the Johns Hopkins Sleep Disorders Center in Baltimore.

DIAGNOSIS AND TREATMENT OF RLS

Because of the unique symptoms that accompany the condition, RLS is often diagnosed simply by the patients' description of the symptoms. If you have the sensation of worms or insects crawling inside your legs that is relieved only when you move or massage your legs, you may have RLS. It is a good idea to see a sleep specialist, who can give you a physical exam that will rule out the possibility of other conditions.

The American Sleep Disorders Association suggests that some home remedies are effective in the relief of RLS symptoms. These include a hot bath, leg massages, a heating pad, ice packs, aspirin or other pain relievers, regular exercise, and the elimination of caffeine. Your physician may also prescribe medication.

It is interesting to note that although Periodic Limb Movement Disorder/PLMD (see Section 42) and RLS are two different disorders, about 80 percent of those who have RLS also have PLMD, but only 30 percent of those with PLMD also have RLS. Many of those with PLMD and/or RLS are tired during the day because they wake from sleep so often during the night; this can lead to a misdiagnosis of insomnia.

For further information about restless leg syndrome, contact the Restless Leg Syndrome Foundation, listed in Section 50.

#44

Rule Out SAD

Some people react to the shortened daylight hours during winter with a condition called seasonal affect disorder (SAD). It is suspected that the lack of bright light on winter mornings delays the body's ability to reduce production of the hormone melatonin (which is produced by the body at night and is tied to sleepiness). The symptoms of SAD appear in the late fall or early winter and last until the following spring.

These light-sensitive people develop feelings of fatigue and drowsiness, and tend to sleep much more than usual during the winter months. Feelings of sadness, irritability, and anxiety accompany SAD, and lack of concentration and social withdrawal often occur. Many develop a craving for carbohydrates such as potatoes, bread, rice, and pasta. There is also an increase in nighttime waking insomnia and a lighter, restless sleep underlies the daytime sleepiness; these symptoms cause some to confuse SAD with insomnia.

Bright-light therapy (see Section 39) is particularly effective in treating SAD. The artificial light changes the production schedule of melatonin and restores the natural feelings of alertness in the morning.

SAD tends to run in families. Women are affected more often than men. Most cases occur in people in their twenties through forties. All people experiencing SAD have one thing in common: When the days grow longer, the condition disappears. Many find themselves supercharged with energy and happiness in the spring and summer.

#45

CONSIDER OTHER
PARASOMNIAS

There are three other fairly common sleep disorders that often are mentioned in discussions of insomnia—night terrors, sleepwalking, and seasonal affect disorder. Before you decide that you have insomnia, first rule out these sleep problems.

NIGHT TERRORS

Night terrors are more commonly found in children than adults. About three to four percent of all children experience this nighttime disturbance. Although the majority of affected children are male and occurrences most commonly peak around age three and disappear by age five, females are not immune and cases have been reported in children from ages six months to thirteen years and beyond.

In a typical night-terror scenario, a parent hears a cry in the dark. She rushes to the bedroom to find her child running around the room crying in terror. You try to stop him and assure him everything is all right. But he pulls away, yells out jumbled words, and with eyes wide open but glassy and unfocused, he continues to cry and thrash about wildly. His breathing is rapid and shallow, and his heart is pounding. You can't stop him, and nothing you do consoles him. Then he returns to bed and sleeps soundly.

Although the term night terrors is meant to describe what the child appears to be experiencing, because he has no recollection of the episode in the morning, it more aptly describes how parents feel when they watch their children act as if possessed by some unseen force. They may even think the child is awake and running around, unable to sleep. But in fact the child is sound asleep.

Night terrors have several consistent identifying characteristics. They tend to occur in non-dream sleep states about ninety minutes after the child first falls asleep; on occasion they may occur once more three to four hours later. Typical episodes last less than fifteen minutes, but some stretch to a full half hour. It is very difficult to awaken children during a night terror, and if awakened they appear disoriented and confused. During the night terror their eyes are open but look glassy and unfocused; the children are not aware of anyone else in the room and aggressively resist being comforted or held. In mild cases they don't cry out but perform repetitive acts such as picking at their pillow or thrashing about in their bed. In severe cases the child jumps out of bed and runs around the room as if in panic. Most mumble or cry out incoherent phrases, but some may yell out statements such as "He's going to get me!" as if in fear of attack.

In most cases night terrors decrease in frequency and duration as children mature. In one study researchers found that affected children who were younger than three and a half years old experienced approximately one episode per week, and these occurrences diminished to one to two episodes per month when they passed the age of three and a half. On the other hand, these researchers found that when children were over three and a half when they experienced their first night terror, the frequency and duration of the following episodes were more severe.

Dr. Charles Schaefer, director of the Sleep Disorders Clinic at Fairleigh Dickenson University in New Jersey, assures us that most childhood night terrors are not caused by psychological trauma. "In fact," he says, "children experiencing night terrors are consistently found to be perfectly normal. They show no signs of abnormal behavior, abnormal psychological profiles, or abnormal brain activity as recorded on electro encephalograms." In addition, personality and behavioral tests have not been able to isolate a particular "type" of child who is likely to be afflicted by these night frights. In any apparent psychological and physical ways, children who suffer through night terrors are no different from other children.

SLEEPWALKING

In the movies, the sleepwalker holds his arms out straight in front and walks as if drawn by a magnet, with stiff, steady legs toward a definite goal. But this image doesn't at all match the reality of sleepwalking, in which people appear to be wide awake and acting quite normally. Although not really awake, sleepwalkers have been known to turn on lights, use the bathroom, change clothes, eat a meal, and even go for a walk or a drive in a car. One way to distinguish sleepwalking from insomnia is to question if the person remembers the episode the following day. An insomniac will remember watching TV at two in the morning; a sleepwalker will not.

Sleepwalking (also called somnambulism) occurs as a person starts to make the transition from a deep-sleep state (stage three) to the lighter-sleep dream state of rapid eye movement. The fact that sleepwalking happens while the sleeper is not yet dreaming negates the age-old belief that a sleepwalker is acting out a dream. Although the exact reasons for sleepwalking are difficult to pinpoint, researchers do know that the causes vary according to the sleeper's age.

In children, sleepwalking is usually a benign problem that is eventually outgrown. It is a part of maturation that affects fifteen percent of all children ages five to twelve at least once. If the first occurrence appears before age ten, it is usually outgrown before age fifteen. Only about two percent continue to sleepwalk as adults.

In adults, sleepwalking is likely to be symptomatic of a psychological or medical disorder. Although adults who sleep-walk are often predisposed to the disorder through genetic or maturational factors, episodes are most likely to occur and to increase in frequency when the adult is feeling highly stressed or is on certain medications that are known to disrupt the sleep cycle.

In the elderly, sleepwalking is usually an indication of an organic brain syndrome frequently called "nocturnal waking." Because there is a progressive decrease in sleep stages three and four throughout life, with a virtual absence of stage four, the onset of sleepwalking episodes similar to those in children or young adults is extremely uncommon in older people. Instead, the most common cause of sleepwalking in the elderly is nocturnal delirium. These episodes often occur in patients with mild or moderate dementia who may function fairly well in the daytime but get up and roam the house at night.

If sleepwalking occurs only occasionally and the person shows no sign of emotional disturbance during the episode, the best course of action is to stop worrying about the act itself and concentrate instead on ways to protect the sleep-walker from harm. You might hide the car keys at night, put away dangerous objects, safety-proof the bedroom, block the doorway, and set alarms to alert bed partners if the doors to the house are opened.

If sleepwalking experiences are frequent (two or three times a night) or intense (accompanied by signs of extreme agitation), or if the sleepwalking puts an individual at high risk of injury, you should seek professional help.

CHAPTER EIGHT

STAY INFORMED

#46

Keep Up on the Latest

Insomnia research is ongoing all over the world. New discoveries, insights, and remedies not mentioned in this book will continue to be developed and will become experimental or standard practice in the treatment of insomnia. The following are just a few studies underway that give us a hint of what's on the horizon.

The Slumber Switch

Harvard researchers have found what they call a "slumber switch" buried in the brain. Scientists hope that this discovery of a process that slips an alert mind into deep and restful sleep may lead to drugs that will end the sleepless nights of insomnia.

In experiments with rats, brain researchers found that during sleep most of the nerve cells of the brain are turned off by a signal sent out by a group of cells in the hypothalamus. Dr. Clifford Saper, chief neurologist at Beth Israel Hospital in Boston and a professor at Harvard Medical School, explains it this way: "To produce natural sleep, you need to turn on these cells. If drugs could be found to activate the cells, then normal sleep could be promoted with pills that have no hangover effects."

The Harvard studies used biological markers to track the activity of rat brain cells during sleep. It was found that this area was the only neuronal structure in the brain that becomes very active during sleep. "As soon as the animal goes to sleep, everything turns off in the brain except for this one little cell group, and it turns on," Saper said.

The precise chemistry of what prompts the nerve cells to act and how the brain overcomes this effect when it awakens are not known, but Dr. Saper said additional experiments with laboratory animals may provide the answers.

This study was reported on January 12, 1996, in *Science*, the journal of the American Association for the Advancement of Science.

A MOLECULE OF SLEEPINESS

Sleep scientist Steven J. Henrikson and his team at the Scripps Research Institute in La Jolla, California, have found a compound in sleepy cats that may be the long-sought substance that could bring natural, drug-free sleep with no hangovers to millions of insomniacs.

This first step used very sleepy cats to unravel, at a genetic and protein level, how sleep works. Henrikson said scientists put the cats on a moving treadmill and deprived them of sleep for up to eighteen hours. Samples of spinal fluid were then removed from the cats, and the chemistry of the specimens was compared to spinal fluid taken from rested cats.

A molecule called cis-9, 10-octadecenoamide was found in the cerebrospinal fluid of sleep-deprived cats. This molecule is known to exist naturally in cats, rats, and humans, and is part of a newly recognized family of brain lipids known as primary amides. A synthetic copy of the molecule was injected into rats; it put them promptly into a deep but natural (not drugged) sleep, demonstrating that the effect works across species. The rats exhibited brain waves associated with normal sleep, reacted instantly to loud noises, and woke up seeming alert and refreshed.

Benjamin F. Cravatt, one of six neuroscientists and chemists at the Scripps Research Institute who reported the findings in a recent issue of *Science*, believes the molecule could possibly be developed into a pill that would bring sleep to the sleepless without causing the next-day symptoms of grogginess, headache, and exhaustion that some experience with sleep medications now in use.

NIGHTCAP

In the January 1995 issue of *Psychophysiology*, sleep researchers Ajilors, Stickgold, Rittenhouse, and Hobson described the first field tests of a home-based sleep-monitoring system called the Nightcap. This sleep-monitoring device uses eyelid and body movement sensors to discriminate awakeness, NREM, and REM sleep automatically. There are already polysomnographic devices that serve this function, but this is the first time the results were able to be gathered in the patient's own home rather than in a sleep laboratory.

The researchers found that the Nightcap is sensitive to clinically relevant changes in the quality of sleep. This new device will prove useful to researchers who want to study sleep in a more natural and cost-effective environment than is possible in traditional sleep laboratories. It also will make the diagnosis of sleep disorders more convenient and comfortable for patients.

If you want to keep up on the latest, be sure to read Sections 47 and 48; they will tell you where to look.

47

READ MEDICAL RESEARCH

If you really want to take a proactive stance and investigate the latest on sleep disorders, a number of resources can help you. Your local reference librarian is probably the best place to start. He can guide you through the various print and computer sources.

Reference librarian Cynthia Hetherington, M.L.S., has mapped out the following sources. Your librarian may recommend others, but these will give you a good start.

PROFESSIONAL ORGANIZATIONS

A good place to start is with the professional organizations that distribute up-to-date information on insomnia. You can find a complete listing in the reference book *The Encyclopedia of Associations*. You can find associations listed under the topic of Insomnia, but keep in mind other terms that may be helpful too, like Sleep Disorders. There are a number of associations listed in Section 50.

On the Shelf

Use the card or computer catalog to find out which books are available through the library. Many libraries are hooked up to a cooperative network of libraries, so even if a book is not immediately available from your own library, it can be ordered for you from another one.

Books in Print

Use the reference books *Books in Print* and *Forthcoming Books* to find out what's been written on the subject of insomnia. If the books you find can't be borrowed through the library, call your local bookstore. They may have some books about insomnia on their shelves, but more valuable is the fact that they can order any book that's still in print right from the publisher.

Medical Reference Books

Your library has a reference section set aside specifically for medical books. Here you'll find medical dictionaries and encyclopedias that may be helpful.

Databases

A good medical database is Medline. Large public libraries and most college libraries subscribe to this information base. Here you'll find a comprehensive and continually updated collection of the latest research on insomnia reported in medical journals. There are other medical databases such as InfoTrac's Health Reference Center that your library may have available.

Your library may also have a database of local newspapers. The health and science sections of many papers run stories on the latest, news-breaking medical studies. You can run a search for any article that discussed Insomnia.

#48

Get On-line

There is a wealth of information regarding insomnia on-line. In a key word search index such as Yahoo, Web Crawler, or Excite, you can search for information sources. To get going, try these:

1. http://sleepnet.com/links.html
   Offers a plethora of information and leads to other Internet sites dealing with sleep disorders
2. http://umt.umt.edu:700/0/general/sleep.txt
   Do's and Don't's for Poor Sleepers
3. http://www.cloud9.net/therapy/
   Sleep Medicine Homepage
4. http://indy.radiology.uiowa.edu/Providers/Publications/AmericanFamily/January1995/Insomnia.htm1
   What to do when you can't sleep: newsletter

5. http://www.social.com/health/nhic/hr2000/
    hr2093.html
    American Sleep Disorder Clinic

Listserves

Listserves, or mailing lists, are forums on the Internet where people can discuss single particular topics. You join through e-mail and participate in moderated discussions that are of interest to you.

Send e-mail to:

listserv@vm.utcc.utoronto.ca

Put nothing in the subject line. In the body type:

subscribe Sleep-L your name

An automated message should respond quickly with further instructions.

(These links are subject to change.)

The National Center for Sleep Disorders Research is on-line and offers information and tips. You can also communicate on SleepL with doctors and researchers in the field of insomnia as well as with other insomniacs.

#49

Investigate
Sleep-Disorders Centers

Looking for the root of insomnia can be a tiring process of elimination. One insomniac may find relief after giving up sleeping pills. Another may finally rest easy after reducing caffeine or nicotine intake. Others find the solution in practicing relaxation techniques. The list goes on and on as discussed in each section of this book. But if your sleep problem doesn't respond to any of these self-help strategies, you may need the kind of specialized diagnostic evaluation offered by sleep-disorders centers. Most of the 298 sleep-disorders centers accredited by the Association of Sleep Disorders Centers offer diagnostic services only, not long-term treatment.

What Happens at a Sleep-Disorders Center?

A sleep-disorders center provides a clinical approach to the diagnosis of sleep problems by monitoring the occurrence of sleep and wakefulness at the time when the problem actually occurs—during sleep. This direct monitoring usually requires no more than a single twenty-four-hour period. Most sleep problems can be sufficiently evaluated with three to four hours of nocturnal sleep. The rest of the time is spent getting an up-to-date record of symptoms and of all the tests that have already been done. Physicians at the center will examine the patient and will generally order additional laboratory tests. Depending on the tests needed and the center's schedule, these may require one or more visits to the center.

After all the data are gathered and evaluated, the patient may be scheduled for one or more polysomnographic recordings. Polysomnography means electrographic monitoring of things like heart activity, brain waves, eye movements, and activity of certain skeletal muscles. Often other tests are added to record respiratory airflow, respiratory effort, oxygen saturation of arterial blood, or erectile activity of the penis.

Depending on the particular problems, polysomnographic recordings may be made during nighttime sleep, daytime sleep, and/or during certain performance tests while awake. The monitoring process begins as sensors are attached to various points on the body about two hours before the intended bedtime. The patient is then put to bed so the functioning of the sensors can be checked. She is told to get as comfortable a night's sleep as possible. The patient can move about freely in bed, and wires can be unplugged easily to permit going to the bathroom.

This monitoring process is painless and rarely prevents sleep. The sleep specialists are aware that the sleep during a clinic visit is not the same as sleep at home, but it is not necessary to have a normal night's sleep to gain the needed information.

Reviewing the polysomnographic data and the historical and psychological data sometimes takes a week to ten days. The patient is usually asked to return to the center for a thorough explanation of what was found. At this time the patient either begins a therapeutic trial to stabilize the symptoms and/or confirm the diagnosis, or is referred back to the primary-care physician with a detailed set of treatment recommendations. The centers remain available for consultation and follow-up.

Is This for You?

Because diagnostic evaluation can be costly and reaching a center may require traveling some distance, take some time to decide if you are an appropriate candidate for sleep-center diagnosis.

Almost everyone experiences occasional sleep problems such as difficulty in falling asleep, many nighttime awakenings, or early morning rising. These are not problems handled by sleep-disorders centers unless they become chronic. Dr. Dement, director of the Sleep Research Center at Stanford University School of Medicine, says that as a flexible rule of thumb, "chronic" means a person who complains of or is impaired by sleep-related problems lasting for more than one month despite compliance with a primary-care physician's recommendations. (Dr. Dement cautions that this rule does not, of course, hold for someone who complains of awakenings at night with palpitation or respiratory crisis that may be a sign of sleep apnea; these should receive immediate attention.)

Sleep problems caused by tolerance to or dependence on sleeping medications are not generally referred to sleep-disorders centers; in these cases withdrawal and detoxification under medical supervision is the recommended course of treatment. But other chronic sleep problems that do not respond to self-help treatments are handled at sleep-disorders centers. These include irregular sleeping schedules and sleep-induced neuromuscular and respiratory problems. Evidence of loud snoring and irregular breathing at night, arrhythmias on the ECG during sleep, and low normal or abnormal blood gases on a pulmonary function test are all ample grounds for seeking a thorough evaluation at a sleep-disorders center.

For Example

In their study, "Sleep Disorders Centers—For Which Patients?" Drs. Dement and Merrill M. Mitler offer two interesting patient scenarios. First they tell of a forty-six-year-old married woman who was seen at a center for a long-standing problem of inability to fall asleep, and frequent awakenings when she did sleep. This problem had grown worse in the past seven or eight months. The patient had tried numerous medications with little effect. Her history did not suggest respiratory or upper airway problems, but she reported that she experienced leg jerks at the onset of sleep. Her husband confirmed this. A psychiatric interview indicated depression, and the patient was tentatively diagnosed as having insomnia secondary to depression.

A nocturnal polysomnogram done in the sleep laboratory disclosed a highly abnormal sleep structure, with rhythmic leg twitches at a rate of three per minute through the first two-thirds of the night. Twitches occurred in groups, ending in arousal or some other disruption of the sleep cycle. The patient was consequently diagnosed as having insomnia associated with nocturnal myoclonus, a diagnosis that would have been impossible without equipment available in a sleep laboratory.

A more common story is told in the case of a twenty-seven-year-old married woman who was referred to a center because she had suddenly begun suffering insomnia at a time when she was experiencing stress and mild depression related to her work. She had been treated with a tranquilizer and an antidepressant, which did not help her sleep problem. Psychiatric examination revealed no contributory difficulties, nor did the medical history and review of systems. However, the interview showed that the patient was very irregular in her going-to-bed times. There was no need to monitor her sleep to discover this problem.

The patient was started on rigorous-schedule therapy, stressing a regular morning arousal time throughout the week, regardless of how long she slept. She was also advised to eat, nap, and exercise at regular times.

At follow-up evaluation after four weeks, the patient reported much less sleep difficulty. She said she no longer worried about an occasional bad night because, with a regular getting-up time, she knew she would be sleepy enough to sleep well the next night.

These two cases give you an idea of the appropriate use of sleep-disorders centers. If all other self-help treatments have failed, talk to your primary-care physician about a referral to a center in your area, or contact the National Sleep Foundation, listed in Section 50.

#50

Contact Associations

As you search for answers, be sure to contact the national organizations who can help you. The groups listed below are a good place to start.

For More Information on Insomnia

American Sleep Disorders Association
1610 14th Street NW
Suite 300
Rochester, MN 55901
507-287-6006

Better Sleep Council
333 Commerce Street
Alexandria, VA 22314
703-683-8371

National Sleep Foundation
1367 Connecticut Avenue NW
Suite 200
Washington, DC 20036
202-785-2300

(This organization can provide you with a list of accredited sleep centers. Be sure to also ask for their bro-
chure "ABCs of ZZZs.")

FOR REFERRALS AND PATIENT SUPPORT GROUPS

Alcoholics Anonymous World Services
475 Riverside Drive
New York, NY 10115
212-870-3400

American Chiropractic Association
1701 Clarendon Boulevard
Arlington, VA 22209
703-276-8800

American Lung Association
1740 Broadway
New York, NY 10019
1-800-586-4872

American Massage Therapy Association
1130 West North Shore Avenue
Chicago, IL 60626
312-761-2682

American Narcolepsy Association
P.O. Box 42460
Cincinnati, OH 45242
513-891-3522

American Sleep Apnea Association
2025 Pennsylvania Avenue NW
Suite 905
Washington, DC 20006
202-293-3650

Depression and Related Affective Disorders Association
Meyer 3-181
600 North Wolfe Street
Baltimore, MD 21287-7381
202-955-5800

National Center for Homeopathy
801 North Fairfax
Suite 306
Alexandria, VA 22314
703-548-7790

National Commission for the Certification of
Acupuncturists
(NCAA)
P.O. Box 9097075
Washington, DC 20090-7075
202-232-1404

Nurse Healers Professional Associates, Inc.
P.O. Box 444
Allison Park, PA 15105-0444

You can leave a voice-mail message by calling
412-355-8476.

Restless Leg Syndrome Foundation
514 Daniels Street
Box 314
Raleigh, NC 27605
919-834-0821

INDEX

® PLUME

HEALING AND HEALTH

☐ **A GYNECOLOGISTS SECOND OPINION** *The Questions and Answers You Need to Take Charge of Your Health* **by William H. Parker, M.D., with Rachel L. Parker and Contributions by Ingrid A. Rodi, M.D., and Amy E. Rosenman, M.D.** Filled with personal accounts from women, this guide answers all the questions women ask about their reproductive system with the most up-to-date medical facts. (276748—$13.95)

☐ **DR. LYNCH'S HOLISTIC SELF-HEALTH PROGRAM** *Three Months to Total Well-Being* **by James P.B. Lynch, D.C., with Anita Weil Bell.** This book will teach you how to use your inner healing force to love and nurture yourself to total well-being. "Dr. Lynch's program is one of self-empowerment. . . . It provides specific steps and self-help tips . . . allowing readers to activate their own natural healing powers."—*Milwaukee Journal* (271509—$11.95)

☐ **PRESCRIPTION OF LONGEVITY** *Eating Right for a Long Life* **by James Scala, Ph.D.** Designed to be fine-tuned to individual needs, this safe, balanced, medically approved diet outlines the ways you can significantly increase your life expectancy—and the quality of your health—simply by altering what you eat. "A fantastic book . . . a 'must read' for every American."—Bruce B. Miller, DDS, PC, President, Diet Analysis Center (270030—$10.95)

☐ **LIVING WITH LUPUS** *A Comprehensive Guide to Understanding and Controlling Lupus While Getting On with Your Life* **by Mark Horowitz, M.D., and Marietta Abrams Brill.** For the half-million Americans suffering from lupus, this informative guide tells what lupus is, its causes, and how it is diagnosed and managed. An extensive glossary and resource listing adds to a wealth of material about this affliction. (270561—$11.95)

☐ **THE WOMAN'S HEART BOOK** *The Complete Guide to Keeping Your Heart Healthy and What to Do If Things Go Wrong* **by Frederic J. Pashkow, M.D., and Charlotte Libov. Foreword by Bernadine Healy, M.D.** This complete guide to women's heart disease and heart health covers every aspect of heart care, heart surgery, and the prevention of heart disease. Filled with life-saving facts that include a diet and exercise life-plan. "A good overview for women who want to prevent the worst."—*Longevity* (272122—$11.95)

Prices slightly higher in Canada.

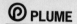